D1447656

Dermatology
Pocket Picture Book

 Barts and The London
Queen

WHITECHAPEL LIBRARY,
020 7882 711

Bo

Dermatology Pocket Picture Book

Anthony du Vivier

Department of Dermatology
King's College Hospital
London

Blackwell
Science

© 2002 by Blackwell Science Ltd
a Blackwell Publishing Company
Blackwell Science, Inc., 350 Main Street, Malden, MA 02148-5018, USA
Osney Mead, Oxford OX2 0EL, UK
Blackwell Science Asia Pty, 54 University Street, Carlton, Victoria 3053, Australia
Blackwell Wissenschafts Verlag, Kurfürstendamm 57, 10707 Berlin, Germany

The right of the Author to be identified as the Author of this Work has been asserted
in accordance with the Copyright, Designs and Patents Act 1988.

All rights reserved. No part of this publication may be reproduced, stored in a retrieval
system, or transmitted, in any form or by any means, electronic, mechanical,
photocopying, recording or otherwise, except as permitted by the UK Copyright,
Designs and Patents Act 1988, without the prior permission of the publisher.

First published 2002

Library of Congress Cataloging-in-Publication Data

du Vivier, Anthony.
    Dermatology pocket picture
  book/Anthony du Vivier.
        p.   cm.
    Includes index.
    ISBN 0-632-05428-X (pbk.)
    1. Dermatology—Handbooks,
manuals, etc.
    2. Dermatology—Atlases.
    3. Skin—Diseases—Handbooks,
manuals, etc.
    4. Skin—Diseases—Atlases.
    I. Title.
    [DNLM: 1. Skin Diseases—Atlases.
WR 17 D987d 2001]
    RL74 D8 2001
    616.5—dc21   2001025449

ISBN 0-632-05428-X

A catalogue record for this title is available from the British Library

Set in 8/10.5 Meridian by SNP Best-set Typesetter Ltd, Hong Kong
Printed and bound in Slovenia by Mladinska knjiga tiskarna d.d.

Commissioning Editor: Stuart Taylor
Editorial Assistant: Geraldine Jeffers
Production Editor: Fiona Pattison
Production Controller: Kate Charman

For further information on Blackwell Science visit our website:
www.blackwell-science.com

SBRLSMD

CLASS MARK   WR17 DER

CIRC TYPE   1 wk

SUPPLIER   CISL   18 3 04
                  £19.95

READING LIST

OLD ED CHECK

Contents

Preface

This small book can easily be slipped into the pocket of a white coat whilst approaching the subject of dermatology. It should serve as an outline of common and important skin disorders and as an *amuse bouche*—a taster—for the greater picture, which is more lavishly illustrated in CD-ROM format (Blackwell Science, 1998) as a bank of 2500 images, of which only a small proportion are reproduced here. In addition, the differential diagnosis of skin eruptions favouring certain sites and of those presenting acutely are tabulated.

Acknowledgements

Most of the patients shown here were treated at King's College, a premier London teaching hospital, with the help of some wonderful dermatological colleagues with whom it has been the greatest pleasure to be associated. They include Andrew Pembroke, Michèle Clement, Barry Monk, Sallie Neill, Pamela Todd, Olivia Schofield, Hywel Williams, Elisabeth Higgins, Noreen Cowley, Jenny Hughes, Claire Fuller, Fiona Child, Fiona Keene, Stephanie Munn, Karen Harman, Lindsay Whittam, Deidre Buckley, Genevieve Osborne, Daniel Creamer, Sarah Macfarlane, Helen Robertshaw, Nuala O'Donaghue, Kate Short and Simon Dawe. The photographs were expertly taken by Barry Pike, Yvonne Bartlett, David Langdon and other members of the Medical Illustrations Department at King's.

I am most grateful for the patience of my Editor, Fiona Pattison, and for the way she has taken care of the project. I would also like to acknowledge Stuart Taylor who masterminded the imagebank on which this book is based and who must be one of the most delightful men in the publishing world to work with.

1 Definitions

A *macule* is a flat lesion less than 1 cm in diameter. The colour of the macule, the presence or absence of changes on its surface and its (or their) whereabouts further aid the diagnosis.

A *patch* is a flat lesion greater than 1 cm in diameter, in other words a large macule, and therefore like a macule may be further described in terms of colour and distribution and also of surface changes.

A *papule* is a raised lesion which is less than 1 cm (some say 0.5 cm) in diameter. A plaque is therefore anything larger than this. Further clarification of the aetiology of the papule(s) may be made by colour, surface and distribution, and whether it is solitary or multiple.

A *nodule* is a raised, solid, palpable mass which is more than 0.5 cm in diameter. It may be due to involvement of the epidermis, the dermis or subcutis either singly or in combination. It may be caused by a developmental fault, inflammation, infection, metabolic disease or neoplasia.

A *plaque* is a slightly raised lesion greater than 1 cm in diameter.

A *vesicle* is a raised lesion containing initially clear fluid which is less than 0.5 cm in diameter.

A *blister* or bulla is a raised lesion greater than 0.5 cm in diameter containing initially clear fluid.

A *pustule* is a raised lesion less than 0.5 cm in diameter containing purulent material which may or may not be sterile.

A *weal* is a transient itchy pink or red swelling of the skin, often with central pallor which disappears without trace. Weals vary in size and shape. The weal is the cardinal physical sign of urticaria. It may be associated with dermographism and angio-oedema. Certain disorders may have an urticarial or urticated component.

An *erosion* is a partial loss of the epithelium. An *ulcer* is a complete loss often accompanied by loss of the dermis and underlying tissues. They are secondary events usually following either a primary blistering process, a vascular event, infection or neoplasia.

Excess or disordered production of keratin may result in *hyperkeratosis*, which is manifest as a roughness, horniness or *wartiness* of the skin.

1

A *crust* is a dried exudate, which may originally have been serous, purulent or haemorrhagic.

Disorders which affect the proper formation of keratin in the stratum corneum of the epidermis may result in *scaling*. Peeling off of the skin is known as *desquamation* and may occur focally or in sheets, secondary usually to a dermal event.

Lichenification is a thickening of the skin with a pronounced exaggeration of the skin creases visible on its surface. It results from rubbing or scratching of the skin either as a primary event, for example lichen simplex, or secondary to an itchy disorder, particularly eczema. Pebbly lichenification is a similar response consisting of flat-topped lichenoid (lichen planus-like) papules.

An *excoriation* is a shallow haemorrhagic excavation of the skin resulting from scratching. It may be linear or punctate. Excoriations may be secondary to a pruritic skin disorder or a systemic disease.

Sclerosis is a diffuse or circumscribed tethering, hardening or induration of the dermis and subcutaneous tissue due to cellular infiltration, collagen proliferation or hyalinization and oedema. It may result in atrophy of the epidermis. It is classically seen in scleroderma or its variants.

Telangiectasia is a dilatation of capillaries. It may be the only physical sign, for example on the face secondary to alcohol misuse, or it may accompany other abnormalities.

Atrophy is a thinning, wrinkling and transparency of the skin due to diminution of one or more elements of the skin, either the epidermis, dermis or subcutaneous tissue.

A *Koebner phenomenon* is the appearance of an eruption in skin subjected to trauma often by scratching but also following a surgical incision, a burn or other injury. Psoriasis, lichen planus, plane warts and vitiligo are the examples of conditions where this may occur.

2 Eczema

Definition

Eczema is an inflammatory disorder of the skin which results in varying degrees of malfunction of the epidermis. It may be acute and vesicular due to intercellular oedema, subacute with less serous exudation, or chronic with thickening of the skin (acanthosis), scaling and excess production of keratin (hyperkeratosis) due to intracellular as well as minor intercellular oedema. These produce different clinical appearances. There is a multiplicity of causes of eczema.

Atopic eczema (dermatitis)

Definition

A chronic pruritic inflammatory disorder affecting the epidermis, commencing in infancy, often persisting throughout childhood but eventually remitting and sometimes recurring in adult life. Genetically determined and associated with other atopic disorders, it is characterized by an imbalance of the immune system with an increase in immunoglobulin E activity and a deficiency of cell-mediated delayed hypersensitivity.

Characteristics

Symptoms
An itching rash.

Signs
Lesions:
• patches (chronic)
• vesiculopapules (subacute) (Fig. 2.1)
• vesicles (acute)
• lichenification (effect of scratching/rubbing) (Fig. 2.5)
• lichenified papules (effect of scratching/rubbing)
• excoriations (effect of scratching/rubbing)
Colour:
• pink
• post-inflammatory hypo- or hyperpigmentation in non-white skin
Surface:
• dry and scaly (chronic) (Fig. 2.2)
• weeping (subacute and acute)
Shape:
• ill-defined

Distribution
Anywhere but especially:
- face
- flexures (Fig. 2.3)

Special features
- associated ichthyosis/xerosis
- keratosis pilaris
- susceptibility to bacterial infection
  —*Staphylococcus aureus*
  —*Streptococcus pyogenes*
- susceptibility to viral infection
  —warts
  —molluscum contagiosum (Fig. 2.4)
  —herpes simplex (Kaposi's varicelliform eruption)
  —vaccinia (formerly following smallpox vaccination)

Variants
- discoid eczema of young adults
- cheiropodopompholyx (idiopathic hand and foot eczema)
- primary irritant eczema of the hands (housewife's dermatitis)
- nail dystrophy

Diagnosis
- clinical
- histopathology (rarely necessary)

Differential diagnosis
Of infantile eczema:
- seborrheic eczema
- scabies
Of childhood eczema:
- scabies
Of adult eczema:
- contact dermatitis
- scabies

Treatment
- emollients
- topical steroids
- impregnated (with tar, zinc, clioquinol, ichthammol) bandages
- antihistamines
- anti-infectives
- tacrolimus
- occasionally oral immunosuppressives

Seborrhoeic eczema of infancy

Definition
A common short-lived non-pruritic inflammatory disorder of the first few weeks of life affecting especially the scalp, face, axillae and napkin area which disappears within 6 weeks.

Characteristics

Symptoms
- usually none
- onset at 4–6 weeks of age

Signs
Lesions: patches.
Colour: pink/red.
Surface: scaly—may be quite thick on the scalp.
Shape: varied due to confluence of the ill-defined patches.

Distribution
- scalp (cradle cap)
- face
- neck, axillae, napkin area
- trunk

Special features
None.

Differential diagnosis
- atopic eczema (Table 2.1)
- napkin eruptions (Fig. 2.7)

Treatment
- emollients
- mild topical steroids

Adult seborrhoeic eczema

Definition
A chronic inflammatory scaling process with a characteristic distribution occurring very commonly on the scalp and face, and less often on the front and back of the chest and occasionally in the axillae and groin.

Characteristics

Symptoms
• cosmetic
• mildly pruritic

Signs
Lesions: scales only or scaly macules or patches.
Colour: pink.
Surface: fine scale, dry.
Shape: ill-defined.

Distribution
Scalp:
• minor non-inflammatory (dandruff)
• inflammatory
Face (Fig. 2.6):
• eyebrows
• sideburns
• eyelids (marginal blepharitis)
• alae nasi
• cheeks
• ears
Torso:
• presternum
• central upper back
Flexures:
• axillae
• groin (Fig. 2.15)

Variants
Annular seborrhoeic eczema.

Diagnosis
• clinical
• rarely skin biopsy

Associations
• stress
• Parkinson's disease
• HIV-related disorders

Differential diagnosis
• scalp conditions
• facial eruptions (especially scaly red patches/plaques)
• flexural rashes (groin/axillae)

Treatment
- imidazole shampoos
- mild topical steroids often combined with imidazoles for face
- moderately potent steroids for flexures
- potent topical steroids for torso
- tar
- lithium succinate and zinc topically
- occasionally systemic imidazoles

Discoid (nummular) eczema

Definition
A morphological description of a form of eczema, predominantly affecting the limbs, which is a distinct entity in the middle-aged and elderly patient and is sometimes associated with alcohol misuse (see Fig. 2.8).

Characteristics

Symptoms
Very itchy.

Signs
Lesions:
- patches
Colour:
- pink
Surface:
- uniformly scaly
- may be acute weeping and crusted or subacute
Shape:
- very well defined
- round

Distribution
Limbs (Fig. 2.8).

Associations
- older age groups
- alcohol and stress

Differential diagnosis
- tinea
- annular lesions

Treatment
- potent or superpotent steroids
- soporific antihistamines at night

Pompholyx (dyshidrotic eczema)

Definition
A pruritic, episodic, sometimes chronic vesicular eruption of the sides of the fingers and toes, and palms and soles associated with hyperhidrosis. It may become dry, fissured and uncomfortable. It is more common in atopics.

Characteristics

Symptoms
Very itchy 'bubbles' under the skin of the palmar or plantar surfaces which weep and then dry and become painful and cracked.

Signs
Lesions: tiny vesicles (Fig. 2.9) which may coalesce and become bullae, then break and ooze serous fluid and subsequently dry when the skin is red, dry, hyperkeratotic and fissured.

Distribution
- sides of the fingers
- palms and soles

Variants
Keratolysis exfoliativa (fine exfoliation due to minor subcorneal blistering).

Associations
- hyperhidrosis
- occasionally an 'id' reaction to a severe tinea pedis

Differential diagnosis
Cheiropompholyx:
- contact dermatitis
- hand eruptions

Podopompholyx:
- tinea
- foot eruptions

Treatment

Acute
• systemic steroids
• soaks (aluminium acetate or potassium permanganate)
• potent or superpotent steroids

Chronic
• potent or superpotent steroids
• emollients

Lichen simplex

Definition
A pruritic eczematous condition resulting from continued rubbing and scratching at a localized area of the skin and often associated with a period of anxiety. It is sometimes chronic.

Characteristics

Symptoms
Itch.

Signs
Lesion: a solitary unilateral plaque.
Colour: flesh-coloured pink hyperpigmented.
Surface: lichenified (Fig. 2.10).
Shape: well defined.

Distribution
Anywhere but especially:
• back of neck
• just below elbow
• back of hand
• genitalia (Fig. 2.11)
• buttock
• lower leg

Special features
None.

Variants
Lichen simplex chronicus.

Diagnosis
- clinical
- biopsy—rarely required, shows eczema

Associations
Anxiety.

Differential diagnosis of lichen simplex chronicus
- any solitary plaque
- hypertrophic lichen planus
- eczema craquelé (Fig. 2.12)

Treatment
Superpotent steroids.

Contact dermatitis

Definition
An eczematous response to either an external irritant (primary irritant dermatitis) or allergen (allergic contact dermatitis). The former is a result of cumulative exposure to an irritant substance and may occur in anyone but particularly in atopics, and the latter is a form of cell-mediated delayed hypersensitivity to an allergen and only occurs in the predisposed.

Characteristics

Symptoms
Itchy, sometimes weeping rash.

Signs
Those of eczema, although often subacute or acute.

Distribution
Anywhere, but the pattern is suggestive of contact with an external agent.

Special features
- keeps recurring
- autosensitization (Fig. 2.13)

Variants
Primary irritant:
- napkin (diaper) dermatitis
- 'housewife's' dermatitis
- asteatotic eczema
- climatic (winter) eczema

Table 2.1 The differences between infantile atopic and seborrhoeic eczema

	Seborrhoeic eczema	Atopic eczema
Onset	Early, before 6 weeks	Approximately at 3 months
Symptoms	Nil	Itchy
Family history	Nil	Positive for atopy
Duration	6 weeks	Chronic
Distribution	Scalp, face, axillae, napkin area	Face and flexures
Site of onset	Scalp (cradle cap)	Face

Allergic contact dermatitis:
- metal
- rubber (Fig. 2.17)
- cosmetics/medicaments (see Table 2.1)
- matches
- plants
- photocontact
- tattoo

Diagnosis
Patch tests (Fig. 2.17).

Differential diagnosis
As for eczema.

Treatment
- identify and stop the irritant or allergen
- appropriate strength topical steroids
- emollients

Varicose (stasis) eczema

Definition
An inflammatory disorder of the skin of the lower legs associated with venous hypertension.

Characteristics

Symptoms
An itchy rash on the legs.

Signs
Lesion: patches.
Colour: pink or red.

Surface: fine scaling, sometimes with excoriations.
Shape: ill-defined, often round.

Distribution
Lower legs, especially around varicosities (Fig. 2.14).

Complications
Contact dermatitis from medicaments.

Associations
Varicose (venous) insufficiency and ulceration.

Differential diagnosis
- discoid eczema
- psoriasis
- tinea
- other eruptions of the lower legs

Management
- of venous insufficiency
- investigation for contact allergens (patch test)
- potent topical steroids
- antibiotics if infected

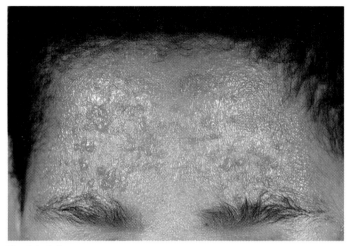

Fig. 2.1 Subacute eczema

Eczema (dermatitis) may be acute, subacute or chronic in morphology. Vesicles and blisters occur in this form but are less pronounced in subacute eczema. The patient observes some degree of weeping of serous fluid from vesicles which forms yellow crusts and may become secondarily infected. This child has atopic eczema.

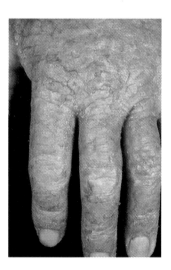

Fig. 2.2 Chronic eczema

In its chronic state the epidermal cells malfunction as a result of intracellular oedema. The epidermis becomes acanthotic (thickened) and the stratum corneum is hyperkeratotic so that the skin is red, dry, scaly, thickened and fissured. These splits in the skin are painful and permit entry of bacteria. Patch tests were negative. This patient had primary irritant dermatitis.

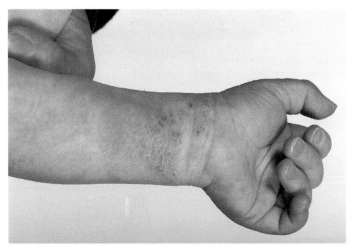

Fig. 2.3 Atopic eczema
By the first birthday the eczema has localized to the flexures, particularly the wrists. The erythema is obvious in white skin but not in black. The patches are ill-defined.

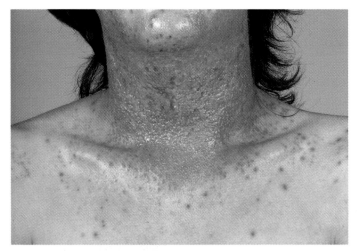

Fig. 2.4 Eczema herpeticum (Kaposi's varicelliform eruption)
Atopics are prone to bacterial (sepsis) and viral infections (especially mollusca and herpes simplex). The individual discrete vesicles on an erythematous surround are clear on the patient's upper chest. On her neck they have coalesced and produced a raw weeping area discharging viral particles. The patient may be very ill with viraemia. The disease had a significant mortality prior to the advent of oral and topical acyclovir.

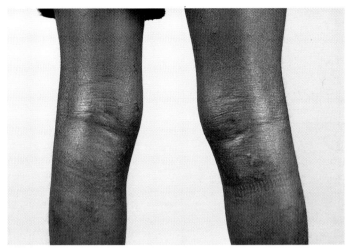

Fig. 2.5 Atopic eczema
Lichenification of the flexures is more obvious as the disorder becomes chronic.

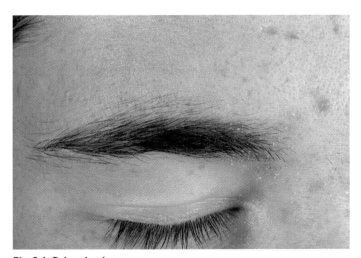

Fig. 2.6 Seborrhoeic eczema
The medial aspect of the eyebrows, the alae nasi and scalp (dandruff) are very commonly affected. There is erythema and scaling and often associated acne vulgaris. The yeast, *Pityrosporom orbiculare*, is associated with the eczema and imidazole shampoos and imidazole combined with hydrocortisone creams may be helpful. The yeast flourishes in immuno-suppressed patients carrying HIV.

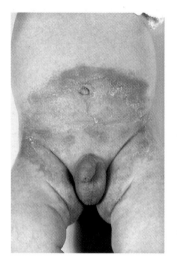

Fig. 2.7 Napkin (diaper) dermatitis
The distribution of the eczema (dermatitis) corresponds to the area of skin covered by the nappy. It is an irritant form of dermatitis resulting from the cumulative insult of urine and faeces on the susceptible skin. In seborrhoeic eczema it spreads beyond this area to the torso, axillae and face.

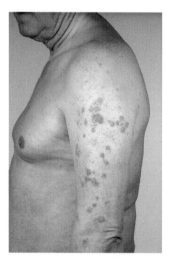

Fig. 2.8 Discoid eczema
The outer aspect of the limbs are particularly affected in discoid eczema but in severe cases it may spread onto the trunk. There are two varieties of discoid eczema. One is associated with atopic eczema, occurs in the young and often results in post-inflammatory hypopigmentation in sunbathers. The other arises in later years, is most common in males and may be a sign of alcohol misuse.

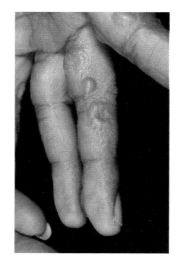

Fig. 2.9 Pompholyx
The palmar and plantar surfaces are affected. Itchy vesicles occur along the sides of the fingers. They subsequently break leaving a raw fissured skin which is pink and scaly. Potent topical steroids are effective but in more acute bullous cases 30 mg prednisolone reduced over 3 weeks may be necessary.

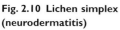

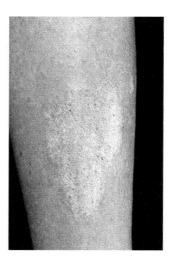

Fig. 2.10 Lichen simplex (neurodermatitis)
The plaque is well defined. The skin is thickened and the skin creases are accentuated (lichenified). It is usually unilateral, which serves to distinguish it from psoriasis. The lateral aspect of the lower leg is a common site. It results from rubbing and scratching of the skin. Superpotent steroids are effective.

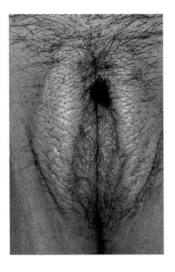

Fig. 2.11 Lichen simplex
The skin is thickened. The skin markings are pronounced. In this case the plaques are bilateral. The condition is entirely secondary to rubbing and scratching the skin. The genitals are a common site.

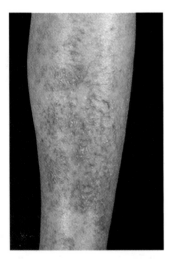

Fig. 2.12 Eczema craquelé
This is common on the lower legs in the elderly. It is often seen after a patient is admitted to hospital for an unrelated condition and results from over-zealous washing of the skin by the nursing staff. The skin on the lower legs tends to be dry anyway in the elderly due to solar damage and hormonal changes. It is occasionally a manifestation of myxoedema.

Fig. 2.13 Contact dermatitis and autosensitization
This patient has an ill-defined patchy red scaly eruption on both her legs. She had developed a contact dermatitis to paraben (a preservative). This was subsequently confirmed on patch testing, when the eruption had been treated. Although she had only been applying the medicament to the legs, the eruption had spread elsewhere as part of a general allergic reaction. This is known as an autosensitization phenomenon.

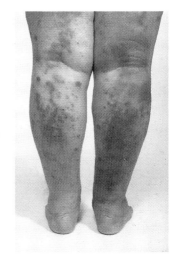

Fig. 2.14 Varicose eczema
There are ill-defined pink patches with a fine scale on the inner leg in association with varicosities. Some are oval and others round. There is a tendency for them to be ill-defined. They are very itchy. These eczematous patches respond to potent topical steroids and measures to combat the venous hypertension and peripheral oedema.

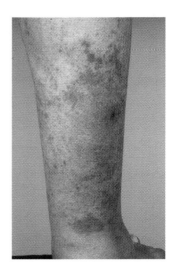

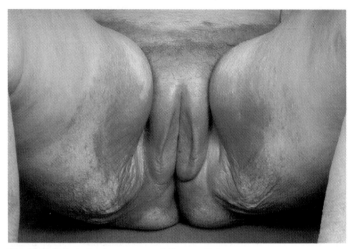

Fig. 2.15 Seborrhoeic eczema of the genital area
There is diffuse ill-defined erythema and scaling. This is an eczema and could also represent contact dermatitis but patch tests were negative. The patient was elderly and presented late but had also been mismanaged by being treated with antifungals. Topical steroids healed it within 72 hours.

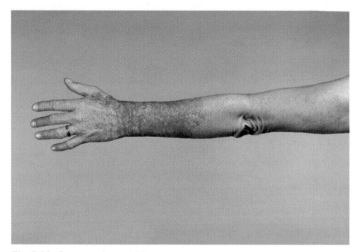

Fig. 2.16 Contact dermatitis
The eczema is often more acute in allergic than in irritant dermatitis so that vesiculation and weeping of the skin is seen. Patch tests demonstrated that this patient was allergic to her rubber gloves.

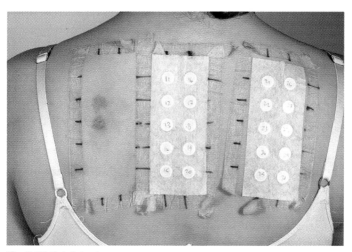

Fig. 2.17 Patch tests

There are approximately 50 substances which are commonly enough
encountered and are responsible for contact dermatitis. This battery of
allergens is applied to the upper back under patches and left in position
for 48 hours and then removed. A positive reaction is a patch of eczema
which is still present 96 hours later. If it has disappeared it is an irritant
effect, not a true allergic one. This eczematous reaction is a manifestation of a type IV delayed hypersensitivity cell-mediated reaction. It is a
permanent allergic state unless modified by the immunological status of
the patient. At present there is no means of desensitizing the patient and
therefore the only means of cure is to avoid exposure to the allergen.

3 Psoriasis

Definition

A common (2% of North Americans and Europeans) benign hyperpro-liferative condition of the epidermis affecting most races but not all (e.g. Indians, but rare in West Indians), and often inherited (autosomal dominant with incomplete penetrance). It presents particularly in adolescence and middle age. It may be associated with nail and joint involvement. It may be precipitated by trauma, stress, alcohol, certain drugs and infections.

Characteristics

Symptoms
Unsightly, occasionally pruritic.

Signs
Lesions: papules which usually coalesce into well-defined plaques (Fig. 3.1).
Colour: red and may result in post-inflammatory hyper- or hypo-pigmentation.
Surface: thick, easily detached white silvery scale with pinpoint bleeding points underneath.
Shape: various, including round and annular.

Distribution
- extensor surfaces, especially elbows, knees, buttocks and scalp
- limbs and trunk
- genitalia
- palms, soles and flexures (less commonly)
- usually spares visible areas such as the face and backs of hands

Special features
- Koebner phenomenon (Fig. 3.2)
- nail involvement (Fig. 3.3)

Variants
- subacute psoriasis
- erythrodermic psoriasis
- guttate psoriasis (Fig. 3.2)
- pustular psoriasis:
  —localized (Fig. 3.4)
  —generalized of von Zumbusch (Fig. 3.5)
- Reiter's disease (Fig. 3.10)

Associations
- seronegative arthritis
- common (5%) in HIV-related disorders
- sometimes associated with alcohol abuse (Fig. 3.6)
- always exacerbated or precipitated by lithium and often by chloroquine or mepacrine

Histology
See Fig. 3.7.

Simulators
Drug eruptions (β-blockers) occasionally.

Differential diagnosis
Not usually a problem for psoriasis vulgaris.
Of scalp psoriasis:
- seborrhoeic dermatitis

Of palmar/plantar psoriasis:
- eczema

Of nail psoriasis:
- tinea

Of guttate psoriasis:
- pityriasis rosea

Of genital psoriasis (Fig. 3.8):
- lichen planus

Treatment

Local
- potent/superpotent topical steroids (not particularly effective and risk of side-effects)
- vitamin D
- tar
- vitamin A
- Dithranol (anthralin) (Fig. 3.9)
- ultraviolet light (very useful, especially narrow band at 310nm)

Systemic
- methotrexate (risk of myelosuppression and liver fibrosis/cirrhosis)
- retinoids (a known teratogen)
- photochemotherapy (PUVA) (a potential skin carcinogen)
- cyclosporin A (side-effects include immunosuppression, hypertension and renal toxicity amongst others)

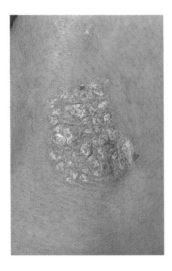

Fig. 3.1 Psoriasis vulgaris
This is a plaque of psoriasis. The disorder is one of benign epidermal cell
hyperproliferation secondary to the
release of polymorphonuclear leuco-
cytes, lymphocytes and lymphokines
from dilated capillaries. A thick,
white, silvery scale and erythema
are therefore prominent features.

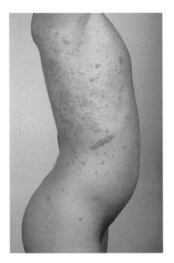

Fig. 3.2 Guttate psoriasis
Guttate psoriasis is an explosive
form of small drops (Latin: *gutta*) or
papules of psoriasis which occurs
approximately 3 weeks after a streptococcal throat infection. It clears
after 4 months, but UVB and tar
baths are good therapy. The
Koebner phenomenon (the appearance of an eruption on skin subjected to trauma) has occurred in a
scratch in this child.

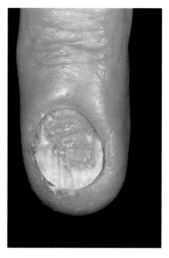

Fig. 3.3 Psoriasis of the nails
Pitting and onycholysis are characteristic of psoriasis. Onycholysis means lifting of the nail away from the nail bed. The nail is white and distally detached. Treatment is limited. Injection of steroids into the posterior nail fold occasionally helps and spontaneous remissions may occur.

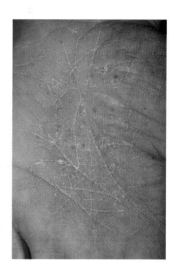

Fig. 3.4 Localized pustular psoriasis
This is usually an intractable chronic disorder of the palms and/or soles. Yellow sterile pustules which turn brown as they resolve occur within a well-defined background of redness and scaling.

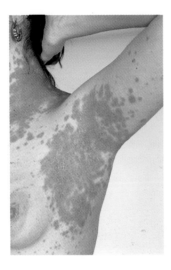

Fig. 3.5 Generalized pustular psoriasis of von Zumbusch
This is an acute sore red pustular form of psoriasis due to an intense invasion of the epidermis by polymorphonuclear cells from the dermis. The pustules are sterile. The patient is ill, feverish and has a leucocytosis. Systemic therapy is indicated.

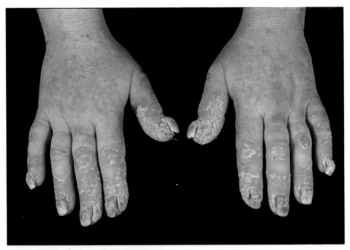

Fig. 3.6 Psoriasis and alcohol abuse
Psoriasis is uncommon on visible sites such as the backs of the hands. There is gross involvement of the nails. This patient was an alcoholic and this acral subacute form of psoriasis is often seen in such patients.

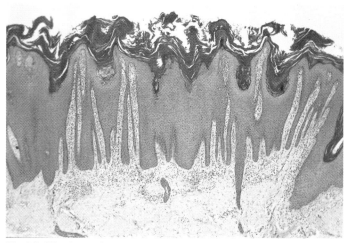

Fig. 3.7 Histology of psoriasis
There is hyperkeratosis and thickening (acanthosis) of the epidermis.
The epidermal ridges are elongated and fused at their lower border.
There are dilated capillaries in the dermis and an infiltrate of poly-
morphs and lymphocytes, which may form aggregations in the epider-
mis known as Munro abscesses.

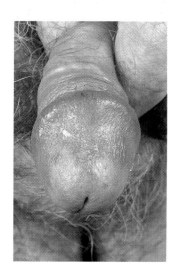

Fig. 3.8 Genital psoriasis
Psoriasis may occur as part of more
generalized disease or in isolation
on the penis although often the
scalp is also involved. There is a
symmetrical red scaling plaque on
the glans.

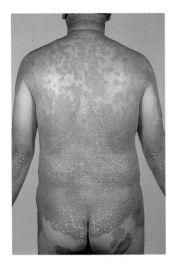

Fig. 3.9 Treatment of psoriasis with dithranol
Dithranol (anthralin) is an effective topical antimitotic agent. It is not easy to use. It may burn the surrounding normal skin and should not be used in the flexures or on the face. It temporarily stains the skin a brown colour. This patient had extensive psoriasis and was treated with dithranol by a nurse in a day-care centre. He also had tar baths and ultraviolet light (Ingram's regime) with complete clearing 5 weeks later. Substantial remissions of 9 months or longer may result. Non-staining derivatives of dithranol (micanol) are available.

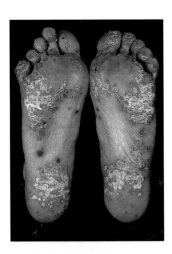

Fig. 3.10 Keratoderma blenorrhagicum in Reiter's disease
The soles are almost always involved a month or two after the arthritis and ocular symptoms. The psoriasiform lesions become heaped up rather like 'a relief map'. The condition is common in AIDS patients who are HLA-B27 antigen positive.

4 Pityriasis Rosea

Definition

A short-lived eruption of unknown aetiology which usually commences as a single oval red scaly 'herald' patch and is followed by a widespread rash composed of similar but smaller patches predominantly on the torso and upper limbs in young people.

Characteristics

Symptoms
Occasionally itchy.

Signs
Lesions: papules initially, which rapidly become patches.
Colour: pink (Fig. 4.1).
Surface: fine scale towards the circumference of the patch.
Shape: oval.

Distribution
• trunk (Fig. 4.2) and upper limbs
• spares face
• more extensive in black skins
• symmetrical

Special features
Herald patch—the first sign of the disorder. It is larger than the subsequent patches. Resolves with a modest degree of post-inflammatory pigmentation in pigmented skin (Fig. 4.3).

Variants

Eczematide—similar morphology but is more extensive and lasts a few months in brown and black skins (Fig. 4.4).
Localized 'sun-spared' pityriasis rosea.

Diagnosis

Clinical biopsy—rarely required; shows eczema.

Differential diagnosis
Herald patch:
• *Tinea corporis* (ringworm)
• any annular patch

The rash:
- secondary syphilis
- guttate psoriasis
- discoid eczema
- pityriasis versicolor
- exanthematic drug eruptions
- any predominantly truncal rash presenting acutely

Treatment
Potent topical steroids.

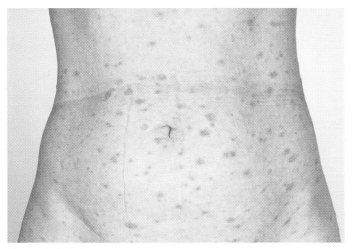

Fig. 4.1 Pityriasis rosea
The pinkness (rosea) of the oval patches and their symmetry is clearly depicted. The condition is common in youth, particularly in the autumn but is not infectious and rarely recurs. It lasts about 6 weeks. Potent topical steroids relieve pruritus if present.

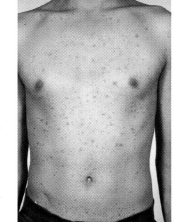

Fig. 4.2 Pityriasis rosea
The pink patches are numerous and by and large symmetrical. The rash spreads rapidly over the body a few days after the appearance of the herald patch. Even if the pink colour is less obvious in a dark skin, the scaliness and oval configuration should aid diagnosis.

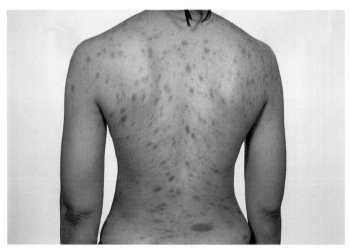

Fig. 4.3 Pityriasis rosea
Occasionally a patient presents after the inflammatory episode has ceased but pigmentation is present. The oval patches and the larger herald patch on her right upper buttock clarifies the diagnosis.

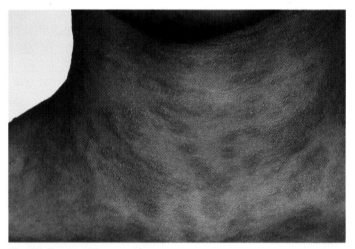

Fig. 4.4 Eczematide
In black people there is an eruption which simulates pityriasis rosea in morphology but is more extensive and lasts several months.

5 Lichen Planus

Definition

A common itchy mucocutaneous disorder affecting all ages and races and both sexes, with a distinctive purple papular morphology and characteristic histology, which persists for a number of months before resolving with temporary post-inflammatory hyperpigmentation.

Characteristics

Symptoms

Very pruritic rash.

Signs (Fig. 5.1)

Lesions: papules which may coalesce into plaques.
Colour: purple.
Surface: flat-topped shiny with reticulate white pattern.
Shape: polygonal.

Distribution

Anywhere, but especially:
• limbs (particularly wrists and ankles)
• lumbar sacral region
• trunk
• umbilicus
• genitalia (Fig. 5.5)

Special features

• Koebner phenomenon (Fig. 5.3)
• resolves with temporary hyperpigmentation (Fig. 5.4)
• oral—white lace-like pattern especially on buccal mucosa (Fig. 5.6)

Variants

• annular
• hypertrophic
• linear
• palmar/plantar
• ulcerative in the mouth
• nail involvement

Diagnosis

• clinical usually
• skin biopsy for histopathology (Fig. 5.2) and sometimes immunofluorescence

Associations
Occasionally:
- diabetes mellitus
- hepatitis C
- primary biliary cirrhosis

Simulators
- drugs
- graft-versus-host reaction
- lichen nitidus

Differential diagnosis
Of common lichen planus:
- scabies
- guttate psoriasis
- lichenoid eczema

Of hypertrophic lichen planus:
- lichen simplex chronicus
- nodular prurigo

Of oral lichen planus:
- oral candidosis

Treatment
Superpotent topical steroids.

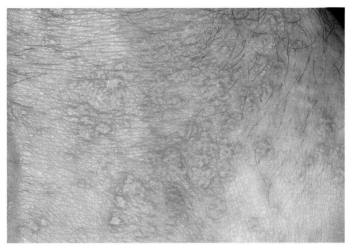

Fig. 5.1 Lichen planus
The purple colour is arresting. The lesions are flat-topped, shiny polygonal papules which may become confluent, forming papules.

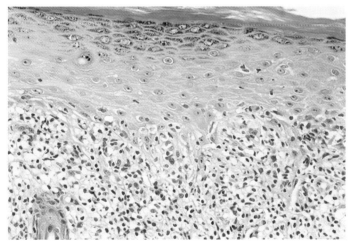

Fig. 5.2 Lichen planus
There is a band-like infiltrate of predominantly lymphocytes with some histiocytes immediately below the epidermis, which destroys the basement membrane and basal cell layer of the epidermis. This produces a saw-toothed appearance.

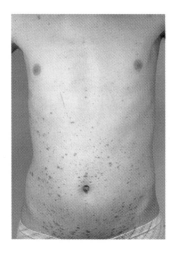

Fig. 5.3 Lichen planus
Multiple purple papules occur. The
disorder affects all age groups and
races. Note the linear Koebner
phenomenon.

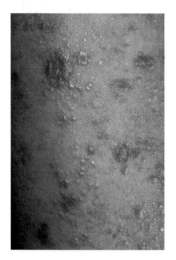

Fig. 5.4 Lichen planus
The shiny active purple lesions are
readily discernible even in pigmented skins. Some have merged
into plaques which become discoloured as they resolve. Post-
inflammatory hyperpigmentation
occurs in all subjects but is most
marked and persistent in brown and
black skin.

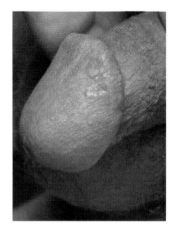

Fig. 5.5 Lichen planus
The glans penis is often involved.
The purple flat-topped papules with
white (Wickham's) striae are clearly
represented here.

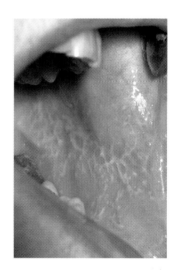

Fig. 5.6 Oral lichen planus
Some of the white papules are discrete and separate but others have
coalesced to produce linear, and in
some areas reticulate, patterns.

6 Naevi

Definition
A naevus is a lesion consisting of one or more of the normal components of the skin. It may or may not be present at birth. The term should be qualified by the name of the cell line involved, e.g. melanocytic naevus, sebaceous naevus, etc.

EPIDERMAL NAEVI

Verrucous epidermal naevus

Definition
A naevus derived from the pluripotential cells of the embryonic ectoderm, specifically the keratinocytes.

Characteristics

Symptoms
A warty lesion usually present from birth.

Signs
Lesions: well-defined papules forming a plaque or plaques.
Colour: pigmented or yellow brown.
Shape: arranged in a linear manner (Fig. 6.1).
Surface: warty (verrucous).

Distribution
- anywhere
- sometimes extensive, often stopping at the midline

Variants
Epidermal naevus syndrome.

Diagnosis
- clinical
- histopathological

Differential diagnosis
- seborrhoeic wart
- warts

Management
Surgical excision if required.

Sebaceous naevus

Definition
A hamartomatous malformation composed of sebaceous glands.

Characteristics

Symptoms
A localized patch which is present at birth and increases in size at puberty. It frequently occurs in the scalp, in which case hair is generally absent.

Signs
Lesions: a plaque.
Colour: yellow.
Shape: oval.
Surface: flat initially but develops small rounded elevations.

Distribution
Head and neck, usually scalp.

Complications
May transform into a basal cell carcinoma (Fig. 6.2).

Diagnosis
• clinical
• histological

Differential diagnosis
• seborrhoeic wart

Management
Surgical excision with primary closure (if necessary after tissue expansion).

Becker's naevus

Definition
A late-onset epidermal naevus with a pigmentary and hairy component most commonly occurring in males.

Characteristics

Symptoms
A large brown mark usually commencing at puberty.

Signs
Lesion: large patch which gradually becomes thickened.
Colour: pigmented.
Shape: irregular.
Surface: often becomes covered with coarse hairs (Fig. 6.3).

Distribution
Usually shoulder or anterior chest.

Management
Possibly lasers.

VASCULAR NAEVI

Strawberry naevi (angiomatous naevi)

Definition
A benign vascular tumour which develops within the first few days or weeks of life and gradually involutes over a number of years. One or several may be present.

Characteristics

Symptoms
A rapidly growing red lump.

Signs
Lesion: a nodule (Fig. 6.4).
Colour: purple or red.
Shape: round.
Surface: smooth.

Distribution
Anywhere.

Progression
Spontaneous resolution within 7 years in the majority of patients.

Variants
Kasabach–Merritt syndrome (a rare haemorrhagic diathesis with thrombocytopenia—due to platelet sequestration and consumption of clotting factors within the angioma).

Management
• reassurance and explanation
• systemic steroids and/or laser therapy if obstruction of breathing, feeding or vision

Port-wine stain (naevus flammeus)

Definition
A permanent purple blemish present at birth often on the face.

Characteristics

Symptoms
A livid birth mark usually on the face.

Signs
Lesion: a unilateral patch.
Colour: red or purple.
Shape: reasonably well defined.
Surface: flat.

Distribution
Usually on the face in the zone supplied by the sensory branches of the trigeminal nerve.

Progression
Permanent.

Associations
Unilateral glaucoma.

Variants
• Sturge–Weber syndrome. The association of a port-wine stain, which is usually but not always more extensive, may cross the midline and extend to the upper eyelid and forehead, with ipsilateral leptomeningeal angiomatosis resulting in epilepsy and contralateral hemiparesis.
• Klippel–Trenaunay–Weber syndrome. The association of a port-wine stain on a limb with increased size of that limb (Fig. 6.5).

Management
• laser therapy
• investigation by CT scanning and magnetic resonance imaging to identify leptomeningeal involvement if indicated clinically

Spider naevus

Definition
A localized punctate arterial dilatation affecting the skin.

Characteristics

Symptoms
A red blemish often on the face.

Signs
Lesion: minute central papule with thin red lines radiating outwards.
Colour: red.
Shape: rather like a spider.
Surface: the lesion may be obliterated by compressing the surface of the central red papule with the wire of a paper clip.

Distribution
Anywhere on the skin in the distribution of the superior vena cava.

Associations
- pregnancy
- oestrogen-containing contraceptives
- liver disease

Treatment
- obliteration with cold point cautery
- lasers

LYMPHATIC NAEVI

Lymphangioma circumscriptum

Definition
A hamartoma of the lymphatic channels resulting in extensive dilatation of the lymphatics in the skin and subcutaneous fat.

Characteristics

Symptoms
Frogspawn-like patches.

Signs
Lesions: vesicles forming numerous and extensive plaques (Fig. 6.6).
Colour: clear or haemorrhagic fluid.
Shape: varied.
Surface: smooth.

Distribution
Predominantly unilateral overlying the buttock, shoulder, perineum or inside the mouth.

Management
Nil (too extensive for effective surgery).

MELANOCYTIC NAEVI (MOLES)

A benign collection of melanocytes which are either present at birth (congenital naevi) or acquired, being located at the dermoepidermal junction (junctional naevi) from whence some (compound naevi) or all (intradermal naevi) migrate into the dermis. They arise from the neural crest early in life. If they are arrested in the dermis *en route* for the epidermis they may be acquired (blue naevi) or congenital (Mongolian blue spot or naevus of Ota). They are often all referred to loosely as moles or birth marks.

Congenital melanocytic naevus

Characteristics

Symptoms
A pigmented birth mark of variable size but always larger than acquired moles (Fig. 6.7).

Signs
Lesion: a flat uniform pigmented patch which may be spotted (naevus spilus) (Fig. 6.8).
Colour: brown, may be *café au lait* in colour.
Shape: oval or round.
Surface: may become thickened and hairy.

Distribution
Anywhere.

Variant
Giant bathing trunk naevus.

Differential diagnosis
See Table 6.1.

Management
• reassurance
• sometimes prophylactic excision if cosmetically acceptable

Table 6.1 The salient features of differential diagnosis of moles and melanoma

Congenital	Comparatively large, present at birth (Fig. 6.6).
Junctional	Small flat and dark, often starting in adolescence (Fig. 6.13).
Compound	Raised often particularly centrally. Two toned (Fig. 6.10).
Spitz	Red-brown papule, often starting in childhood (Fig. 6.12).
Intradermal	Flesh-coloured soft papule, particularly on face (Fig. 6.9).
Blue naevus	Blue or blue-black colour (Fig. 6.13).
Superficial spreading melanoma	Actively expanding, often larger, various shades of pigment, irregular outline (Fig. 8.19).
Papular (nodular) melanoma	Growing papule or nodule, very dark or black in colour (Fig. 8.18).

Junctional naevi

Characteristics

Symptoms
A flat dark mole.

Signs
Lesion: a macule.
Colour: dark brown and/or brown: often two toned.
Shape: oval or round.
Surface: flat.

Distribution
Anywhere.

Diagnosis
• clinical
• histopathological

Differential diagnosis
See Table 6.1.

Management
Reassurance, but excision if in doubt.

Intradermal naevus

Characteristics

Symptoms
A flesh-coloured mole.

Signs
Lesion: a soft papule which may be pedunculated.
Colour: flesh-coloured.
Shape: round or oval.
Surface: smooth, sometimes hairy.

Distribution
Anywhere but particularly the face (Fig. 6.9).

Diagnosis
• clinical
• histopathological

Differential diagnosis
See Table 6.1.

Management
• reassurance
• may be shaved off flush to the skin with good cosmetic results

Compound naevus

Characteristics

Symptoms
A raised brown mole.

Signs
Lesion: a soft papule.
Colour: brown or dark brown, usually two toned either darker centrally or peripherally (Fig. 6.10).
Shape: round or oval.
Surface: usually smooth but sometimes mamillated or papillomatous or hairy.

Distribution
Anywhere.

Variants
Halo naevus (Fig. 6.11).

Diagnosis
• clinical
• histopathological

Differential diagnosis

See Table 6.1.

Management

• reassurance
• excision if required

Spitz naevus (juvenile melanoma)

Characteristics

Symptoms

A red–brown mole occurring usually in childhood, which grows rapidly initially.

Signs

Lesion: a soft papule occasionally nodule.
Colour: red or reddish brown (Fig. 6.12).
Shape: round.
Surface: smooth.

Distribution

Anywhere, especially face (particularly cheeks) and legs.

Diagnosis

• sometimes clinical
• usually histopathological

Differential diagnosis

See Table 6.1.

Management

Often surgical excision.

Blue naevus

Characteristics

Symptoms

A dark-blue lesion often causing concern as to its nature.

Signs

Lesion: a soft papule or nodule.
Colour: blue or blue black (Fig. 6.13).

Shape: round.
Surface: smooth.

Distribution
Anywhere, but particularly back of hand or foot, and face.

Diagnosis
- clinical
- histopathological

Differential diagnosis
See Table 6.1.

Management
- reassurance
- excision if required

Mongolian blue spot

Characteristics

Symptoms
A large blue–grey blemish usually on the buttocks of a new-born mongoloid or negroid baby.

Signs
Lesion: a large, usually single diffuse patch.
Colour: slate blue.
Shape: rounded or oval.
Surface: flat and smooth.

Distribution
Lumbosacral region.

Progression
Usually disappears by the age of 7 years.

Differential diagnosis
None.

Treatment
None.

Naevus of Ota

Characteristics

Symptoms
Facial birth mark near and in the eye, appearing in childhood.

Signs
Lesion: a large diffuse patch.
Colour: a deep blue on the skin but brown on the conjunctiva.
Shape: diffuse on the cheek, patchy or geographical on the conjunctivae.
Surface: flat and smooth.

Distribution
Face and eye (Fig 6.14).

Differential diagnosis
Nil.

Treatment
Lasers may be tried.

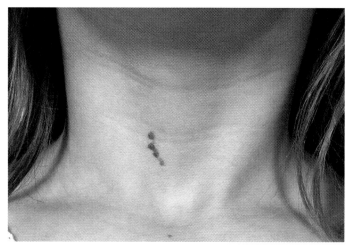

Fig. 6.1 Epidermal naevus

The neck is a common site. The linear pattern is clearly shown. The surface is warty and the yellow/brown colour resembles that of a seborrhoeic wart for which it might be mistaken except that the latter are acquired and not congenital. Surgical excision is the treatment of choice if required.

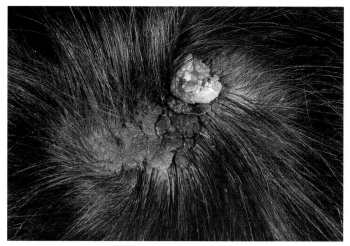

Fig. 6.2 Sebaceous naevus and basal cell carcinoma

There is an increased risk of transformation to a basal cell carcinoma, and the lesion should be excised in its entirety. Many lesions are removed prophylactically for this reason, either by primary excision and closure or by prior use of a tissue expander.

49

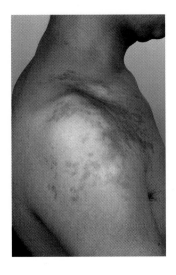

Fig. 6.3 Becker's naevus
The lesion is not present at birth
but usually appears at puberty. It is
flat and pigmented initially and
gradually becomes raised and hairy.
The shoulder is a common site.

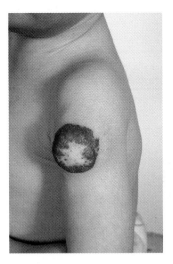

Fig. 6.4 Strawberry naevus
This benign vascular tumour arises
shortly after birth, grows to a
various degree and subsequently
involutes over the next 7 years. It is
of cosmetic significance and does
not require treatment unless the
tumour interferes with feeling or
vision.

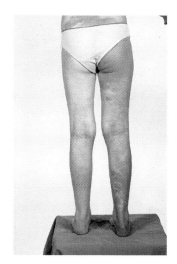

Fig. 6.5 Klippel–Trenaunay–Weber syndrome
This is the association of a port-wine stain and venous varicosities with swelling of the underlying soft tissues and sometimes bone, affecting usually the lower limb.
© Photograph courtesy of Mr Paul Baskerville.

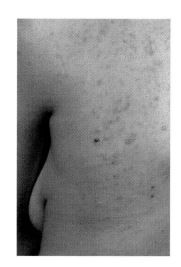

Fig. 6.6 Lymphangioma circumscriptum
There are vesicles forming numerous and extensive plaques. At present surgery is ineffective.

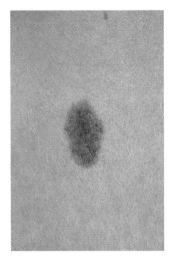

Fig. 6.7 Congenital naevus
This mole was present at birth. About 1% of infants have one. It is larger than an acquired mole, oval in shape and consists essentially of the two shades of brown distributed in a regular and uniform manner. There is a very slightly increased risk of malignant transformation many years later. They should always be protected from the sun.

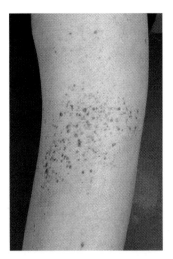

Fig. 6.8 Naevus spilus
This congenital naevus consists of many dark-brown spots (Greek *spilos* = spot) on a light-brown background. It is present at birth.

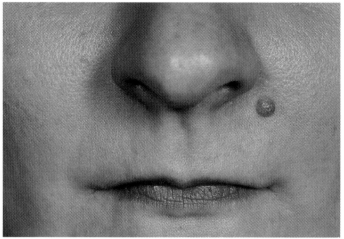

Fig. 6.9 Intradermal naevus
The face is the commonest site and removal is usually requested for cosmetic reasons. They are sometimes called cellular naevi.

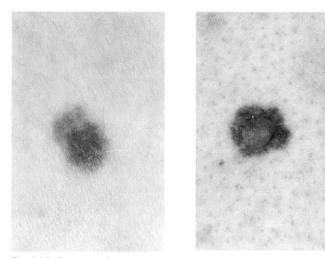

Fig. 6.10 Compound naevus
There are essentially two shades of pigment, brown and light brown, present in this slightly raised mole (left). The arrangement of the pigment is reasonably uniform although not perfectly so. This is often the case. There is a brown soft papule centrally with an even light and dark-brown circumference (right).

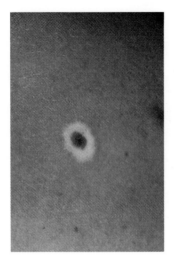

Fig. 6.11 Halo naevus
A white halo of complete loss of pigmentation simulating vitiligo may appear around a compound or junctional naevus. The mole will subsequently disappear and the skin repigment, the process taking some years. It is an autoimmune phenomenon of unknown significance but quite harmless. It may affect multiple naevi and is usually seen in young people.

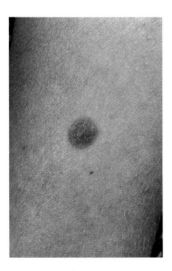

Fig. 6.12 Juvenile melanoma (Spitz naevus)
This occurs most commonly in young people and is often a red/brown papule. The histology may be confused with a malignant melanoma but it is quite benign.

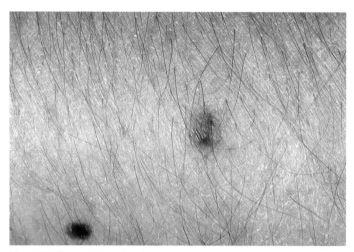

Fig. 6.13 Blue and junctional naevi
The blue naevus on the right should be compared with the brown junctional naevus on the left. The diagnosis is made on the colour. The melanocytes are thought to be halted deep in the dermis during their migration from the neural crest to the dermo-epidermal junction.

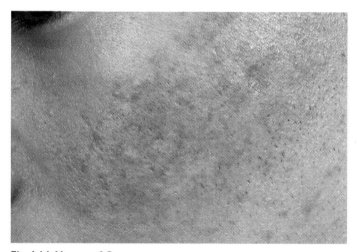

Fig. 6.14 Naevus of Ota
This is most common in Orientals and there is a bluish patch on the cheek, often with involvement of the conjunctiva.

7 Benign Tumours

Cysts

Definition

A swelling in the skin lined histologically by epidermal cells (epidermoid cysts), the external root sheath of the hair follicle (pilar cysts) or sebaceous glands (steatocystoma multiplex). Dermoid cysts arise from epithelium trapped within embryonic fusion lines. Cysts are often, although inaccurately, referred to as sebaceous cysts.

Characteristics

Symptoms
A swelling under the skin.

Signs
Lesion: a nodule.
Colour: flesh-coloured, but may be white or cream-coloured (milia) yellow (steatocystoma multiplex).
Shape: spherical or dome-shaped.
Surface: smooth: may have central keratin-filled punctum (epidermoid).
Size: varies from small (milium) to large.
Consistency: firm, freely mobile within the dermis but tethered to the overlying skin.

Distribution
• especially face, neck and torso (the sites of acne) (epidermoid and sebaceous)
• feet, hands and buttocks (trauma-induced implantation cysts)
• scalp (pilar) (Fig. 7.1)
• embryonic fusion lines (dermoid) presentation at birth or in childhood.
  —outer third of eyebrow
  —midline of nose
  —under chin and front of neck and chest
  —scalp and occiput
  —anogenital area

Complications
• infection
• inflammation
• calcification

Diagnosis
- clinical
- histopathological

Differential diagnosis
Epidermoid cyst:
- central punctum
- greasy, foul smelling contents
- adults

Pilar cyst:
- scalp
- familial

Steatocystoma multiplex:
- yellow, multiple, torso

Dermoid cyst:
- present at birth or in childhood
- specific sites and midline

Associations of epidermoid cysts
- Gardner's syndrome—osteomata, epidermoid cysts and polyposis coli
- Nodulocystic acne

Management
- excision if required
- appropriate antibiotics if infected

Dermatofibroma (histiocytoma, sclerosing angioma)

Definition
A common benign dermal tumour of fibrohistiocytic cells with associated collagen bundle proliferation, present most often on the legs especially in women, possibly the result of a previous insect bite.

Characteristics

Symptoms
One or more unsightly small lumps.

Signs
Lesion: papule and occasionally a nodule.
Colour: red–brown or dark brown (Fig. 7.3).
Shape: round.
Surface: smooth.
Consistency: firm—surface 'dimples' when compressed (Fig. 7.3).

Distribution
Anywhere, especially lower limbs.

Diagnosis
- clinical
- pathological

Differential diagnosis
Papular or nodular melanoma.

Management
Excision if required.

Syringoma

Definition
A developmental disorder of the sweat glands arising in adolescence, particularly in females.

Characteristics

Symptoms
Multiple spots on the face and elsewhere.

Signs (Fig. 7.4)
Lesion: small papules.
Colour: yellow or flesh-coloured.
Shape: round.
Surface: smooth.

Distribution
Characteristically around the eyes and cheeks but also front of the chest and neck.

Diagnosis
- clinical
- histopathological

Differential diagnosis
Milia.

Management
- reassurance
- may be cauterized

Senile sebaceous hyperplasia

Definition
A small benign tumour composed of mature sebaceous glands, usually multiple and common in middle age.

Characteristics

Symptoms
A spot or spots on the face.

Signs
Lesion: papule.
Colour: yellowish.
Shape: round.
Surface: smooth with a central dimple.

Distribution
The face.

Diagnosis
• clinical
• histological

Differential diagnosis
Basal cell carcinoma.

Management
May be destroyed by cautery.

Seborrhoeic wart (basal cell papilloma, seborrhoeic keratosis)

Definition
A very common benign tumour of advancing years composed of a collection of immature keratinocytes and horn cysts in the epidermis.

Characteristics

Symptoms
One or several unsightly 'moles' which may itch.

Signs (Fig. 7.5)
Lesion: papule which becomes a plaque.
Colour: yellow–green or more pigmented.
Shape: well defined.
Surface: rough (warty), fissured and/or stippled.

Distribution
Anywhere, but predominantly areas which have been exposed to sunlight (Fig. 7.2).

Complications
Inflammation.

Differential diagnosis
- superficial spreading malignant melanoma.
- basal cell carcinoma
- Bowen's disease

Management
- cryotherapy
- curettage and cautery if required

Hypertrophic scars and keloids

Definition
Both are a normal hyperproliferative response of connective tissue to trauma. The hypertrophic scar remains confined to the site of the injury and may improve. The keloid spreads well beyond it and is permanent.

Characteristics

Symptoms
An unsightly mark or scar.

Signs
Lesion: a nodule or plaque (Fig. 7.6).
Colour: red–brown, brown or dark brown.
Shape: any.
Surface: smooth.
Consistency: firm.

Distribution
Anywhere, but especially ear lobes, chin, neck, shoulders and upper trunk.

Associations
- familial (5%)
- racial (especially black people)
- surgery in certain areas of the skin
- nodulocystic acne
- folliculitis (nuchal keloids) (Fig. 7.11)
- ingrowing hairs

Management
- difficult
- intralesional triamcinolone for ear lobes and hypertrophic scars
- excision and immediate radiotherapy sometimes effective

Lipoma

Definition
A benign subcutaneous tumour composed of mature fat cells.

Characteristics

Symptoms
A large lump under the skin.

Signs
Lesion: one or several nodules.
Colour: flesh-coloured.
Shape: round.
Surface: smooth, cooler than surrounding skin.
Size: large.
Consistency: soft, lobulated skin overlying the tumour is easily moved.

Distribution
- thighs and upper arms
- neck, shoulders and back

Complications
Very rarely malignant transformation.

Associations
- Gardner's syndrome (osteomata, epidermoid cysts and polyposis coli)
- spina bifida if lipoma in lumbar region
- lipomata of the gut, lungs or genital urinary tract occasionally

Diagnosis
- clinical
- histopathological

Management
Excision only if requested.

Glomus tumour

Definition
A benign painful tumour of the neuromyoarterial glomus apparatus.

Characteristics

Symptoms
A lump which is painful on pressure, in response to temperature changes or spontaneously.

Signs
Lesion: papule or nodule.
Colour: pink or purple.
Shape: round.
Surface: smooth.
Consistency: painful to touch.

Distribution
Extremities or under a nail.

Diagnosis
• clinical
• histopathological

Management
Surgical excision.

Haemangioma and pyogenic granuloma

Definition
A common benign acquired tumour of blood vessels, which if of sudden onset and haemorrhagic is known as a pyogenic granuloma.

Characteristics

Symptoms
A red spot or lump, which may bleed.

Signs
Lesion: papule or nodule (Fig. 7.7).
Colour: bright red (Fig. 7.8).
Shape: round.
Surface: smooth.

Distribution
Haemangioma:
• anywhere

Pyogenic granuloma:
- feet and hands (especially fingers)
- scalp
- upper trunk
- lips

Variants
Campbell de Morgan spots (cherry angiomata).

Diagnosis
- clinical
- histopathological

Differential diagnosis
- amelanotic melanoma

Management
- curettage and cautery (pyogenic granuloma)
- surgical excision if required
- cautery (Campbell de Morgan spots)

Naevoxanthoendothelioma (juvenile xanthogranuloma)

Definition
A benign tumour of non-Langerhan cell histiocytes which occurs in infancy or childhood and resolves spontaneously within 1 or more years.

Characteristics

Symptoms
The appearance of one or several asymptomatic yellow lumps.

Signs
Lesion: papule or nodule.
Colour: yellow.
Shape: round.
Surface: smooth.
Consistency: firm or rubbery.

Distribution
- face, neck and scalp (Fig. 7.9)
- trunk

Associations

- occassionally visceral involvement
- eye involvement quite common
- occasionally neurofibromatosis, juvenile myeloid leukaemia, urticaria pigmentosum

Diagnosis

- clinical
- histopathological

Differential diagnosis

The other common tumours of childhood. The distinguishing features of the common benign tumours of early life are:

Pilomatrixoma:
- a hard lobulated deep nodule

Naevoxanthoendothelioma:
- one or several yellow papules or nodules often around the scalp

Mastocytoma:
- a red–brown plaque which urticates

Juvenile melanoma (Spitz naevus):
- a red–brown papule often on the cheek

Strawberry naevus:
- a substantial red or purple tumour arising within the first few days of life

Management

Reassurance.

Calcifying epithelioma of Malherbe (pilomatrixoma)

Definition

A solitary tumour of the hair follicle which presents early in life.

Characteristics

Symptoms

A single hard lump.

Signs

Lesion: a deep nodule.
Colour: often flesh-coloured or pink (Fig. 7.12).
Shape: round.
Surface: often lobulated.
Consistency: stony hard.

Distribution
Head, neck or upper extremity.

Associations
- very rarely malignant transformation
- with myotonia congenita (unusual)

Diagnosis
- clinical
- histopathological

Differential diagnosis
The other four common childhood tumours. See differential diagnosis for naevoxanthoendothelioma.

Management
Excision.

Mastocytoma

Definition
An accumulation of benign normal mast cells in the dermis, appearing in infancy or childhood and disappearing spontaneously. This is usually solitary.

Characteristics

Symptoms
A red–brown lump which may urticate (itch and develop weals on being rubbed).

Signs
Lesion: a plaque.
Colour: red–brown or orange.
Shape: round.
Surface: smooth.
Consistency: develops a weal and flare or even blister on being rubbed (Fig. 7.10).

Distribution
Anywhere.

Associations
Rarely systemic flushing accompanies local urtication.

Diagnosis
• clinical
• histological (the mast cell granules are stained metachromatically with toluidine blue)

Differential diagnosis
The other common tumours of childhood. See differential diagnosis for naevoxanthoendothelioma.

Management
Reassurance.

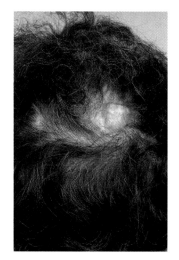

Fig. 7.1 Pilar cyst (trichilemmal cyst)
Often known as 'wens', these are frequently multiple, occur in the scalp and are inherited as an autosomal dominant trait, but are more common in women. They are derived from the external sheath of the hair root.

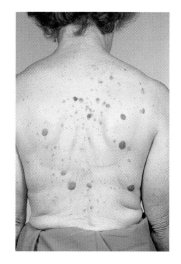

Fig. 7.2 Seborrhoeic warts
Often called 'moles' by patients, they may be numerous. They are quite benign but unsightly and may be removed by curettage and cautery or by cryotherapy. They are sometimes itchy and may become inflamed. They are probably caused by sunburn earlier in life.

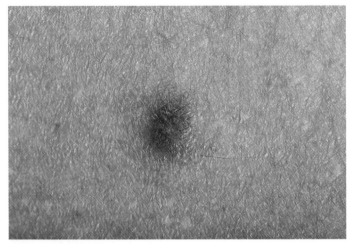

Fig. 7.3 Dermatofibroma
The lesion is a firm red–brown papule most commonly situated on the lower leg and often multiple. It is attached to the overlaying epidermis and wrinkles when compressed between the finger and thumb but is movable within the dermis. They may be secondary to a previous forgotten insect bite. They are most common in women.

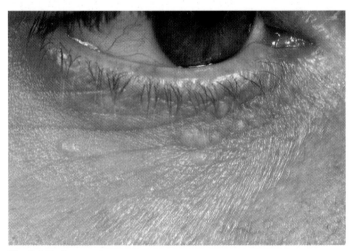

Fig. 7.4 Syringomata
Multiple small flesh-coloured papules are present around the eyes. The site is virtually diagnostic. Histologically there are glandular structures in the dermis some of which are canalized and have a double layer of cells similar to those which line the sweat ducts.

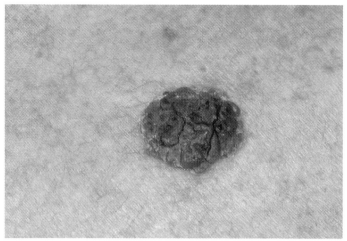

Fig. 7.5 Seborrhoeic wart
This plaque is very well defined. It has a fissured surface. It is a greasy (hence seborrhoeic) yellow–green colour but may be quite heavily pigmented.

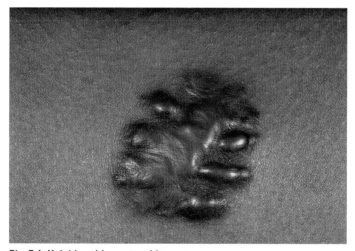

Fig. 7.6 Keloid and hypertrophic scars
The distinction between the keloid and hypertrophic scar is that the former spreads beyond the area of injury whereas the hypertrophic scar does not. Surgery is inadvisable for benign skin lesions in certain sites, which include the front of the chest, upper back and shoulders. A hypertrophic scar is due to abnormal proliferation of connective tissue at the site of the injury and does improve with time. Intralesional triamcinolone may be beneficial in either condition.

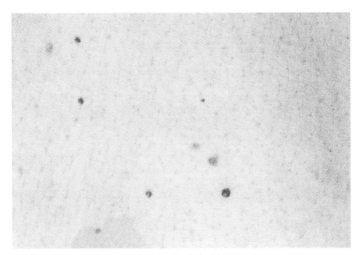

Fig. 7.7 Haemangioma and Campbell de Morgan spots (cherry angiomas)
There is a well-defined smooth-surfaced red papule. They occasionally bleed. They may be multiple and much smaller and appear as bright red macules or papules, which contrast with the brown moles. They are harmless but their cause is unknown.

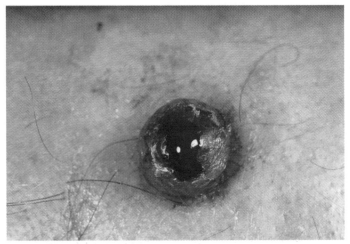

Fig. 7.8 Pyogenic granuloma
This nodule is red–brown in colour. There is evidence of a recent bleed. It grows rapidly initially and then becomes static. It may be removed by curettage and cautery but it may recur.

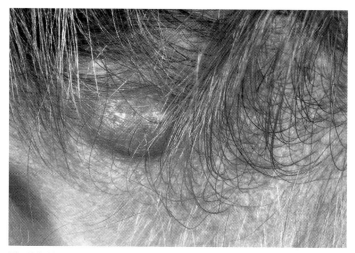

Fig. 7.9 Naevoxanthoendothelioma
There is one or more yellow or orange papules or nodules which arise
in infancy or childhood, persist for a while and then disappear. The head
is the commonest site. It is a benign proliferation of histiocytes.

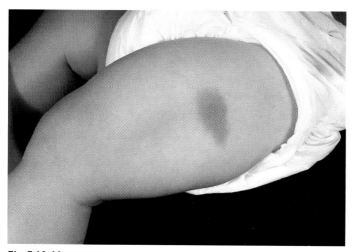

Fig. 7.10 Mastocytoma
The lesion is a red–brown plaque, which reddens, swells and itches with
rubbing. It may even blister. It arises in infancy or early childhood.

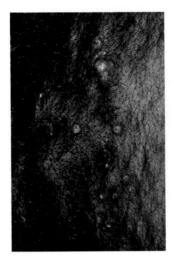

Fig. 7.11 Nuchal keloids
Firm brown papules occur at the nape of the neck in black people secondary to a staphylococcal folliculitis or ingrowing hairs produced by shaving the back of the scalp. They are very difficult to manage, although intralesional steroids may be tried.

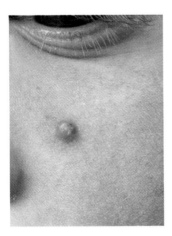

Fig. 7.12 Calcifying epithelioma of Malherbe
Usually seen on the face in childhood it has a hard consistency and has a pink/yellow colour.

8 Skin Cancer

Effects of solar irradiation on the skin

Definition
The development of certain readily identifiable changes in the skin particularly of Caucasians resulting from ultraviolet irradiation.

Characteristics

Symptoms
- sunburn
- in the susceptible phenotype

Signs
- freckles
- lentigines
- seborrhoeic warts
- hypopigmented macules
- white spot disease
- atrophy
- purpura
- scars
- solar elastosis
- cutis rhomboidalis nuchae
- comedones
- milia
- telangiectasia
- poikiloderma of Civatte

Distribution
Light-exposed skin especially:
- face
- hands
- limbs especially lower legs in women
- lips
- scalp
- torso

Actinic keratoses

Definition
A premalignant disorder of the epidermis which may be single or multiple occurring on sunlight-exposed Caucasian skin.

Characteristics

Symptoms
Red rough spot(s) or patch(es) on the face, backs of the hands and/or legs.

Signs
Lesions: papule(s) or patch(es).
Colour: red.
Surface: rough with an adherent scale (Fig. 8.1).

Distribution
- light-exposed skin
- including the mucosa of the lower lip (actinic cheilitis)

Diagnosis
Clinical, but sometimes histopathological.

Differential diagnosis
- psoriasis
- seborrhoeic wart
- viral wart

Treatment
- cryotherapy (liquid nitrogen)
- surgery (usually curettage and cautery)
- topical therapy with 5-fluorouracil (Fig. 8.2)

Bowen's disease

Definition
An intraepidermal carcinoma of the skin which is usually solitary and occurs on sun-damaged skin but occasionally on the genitalia possibly due to wart virus. Multiple lesions may result from previous arsenic ingestion. Bowen's disease may progress to squamous cell carcinoma.

Characteristics

Symptoms
A slowly growing roughened patch.

Signs
Lesions: a patch which becomes thickened forming a plaque (Fig. 8.3).
Colour: red.
Surface: rough with an adherent scale.

Progression (complications)
May thicken further becoming nodular or ulcerated indicating change to a squamous cell carcinoma.

Distribution
Light-exposed skin but especially face, back of the hands or fingers (Fig. 8.4) and lower leg.

Variants
- genital Bowen's disease (Fig. 8.5, 8.6)
- Bowenoid papulosis
- multiple lesions associated with arsenic toxicity

Diagnosis
Histopathology (Fig. 8.7)

Differential diagnosis
- eczema
- psoriasis
- superficial basal cell carcinoma
- seborrhoeic wart

Treatment
- surgical (excision or curettage and cautery)
- cryotherapy
- topical with 5-fluorouracil

Squamous cell carcinoma

Definition
A malignant tumour arising from squamous keratinocytes in the epidermis of the skin or mucous membranes which may eventually metastasize. It usually arises in sun-damaged skin, a solar keratosis or Bowen's disease but may be associated with immunosuppression, X-irradiation, carcinogens such as arsenic and polycyclic hydrocarbons, certain skin disorders and the human papilloma virus.

Characteristics

Symptoms
A crusted growth or ulcer on the skin or mucous membranes which may bleed.

Signs
Lesion: an indurated plaque, nodule or ulcer (Fig. 8.8).
Colour: pink or red.

Surface: crusted and often haemorrhagic, eroded (Fig. 8.9) or ulcerated.
Margin: raised, indurated, heaped up, everted.

Distribution
Light-exposed skin.

Variants and causes (Table 8.1)
• immunosuppression
• X-irradiation (Fig. 8.10)
• certain skin disorders
• photochemotherapy (psoralen + ultraviolet A, PUVA)
• genital squamous cell carcinoma
• epithelioma cuniculatum

Diagnosis
Histopathology

Table 8.1 Causes of squamous cell carcinoma

Irradiation
• ultraviolet light (commonest)
• artificial ultraviolet irradiation including PUVA
• X-irradiation

Immunosuppression following transplant
• especially renal and liver

Human papilloma virus
• especially vulva carcinoma

Chronic scarring conditions
• lupus vulgaris
• lupus erythematosus
• epidermolysis bullosa
• secondary to burns including from erythema ab igne

Mucosal skin disorders
• genital lichen sclerosus et atrophicus (rarely)
• oral or genital lichen planus (very rarely)

Genetic disorders
• albinism
• xeroderma pigmentosum

Exogenous carcinogens
• polycyclic hydrocarbons (e.g. tar, mineral oils, soot)
• arsenic

Differential diagnosis
- keratoacanthoma
- basal cell carcinoma

Treatment
- surgical excision
- radiotherapy

Basal cell carcinoma

Definition
A common malignant tumour derived from the basal cells of the epidermis which is locally destructive but which rarely, if ever, metastasizes. There are a variety of types which occur most commonly on the head and neck and a superficial form, which is found on the trunk or limbs.

Characteristics

Symptoms
A slowly growing painless spot which subsequently bleeds and scabs but never quite seems to heal.

Signs
Lesion: papule which becomes a nodule.
Colour: similar to that of a pearl.
Surface: smooth (cystic) or ulcerated with telangiectasia.
Margin: slightly raised and rolled (all forms except cystic).

Progression (complications)
The lesion is locally invasive and destructive, which is of significance around the eye and the nasolabial and retroauricular folds.

Distribution
- head and neck
- occasionally genital
- limbs and trunk (superficial especially)

Types

Rodent ulcer
Lesion: papule which becomes a nodule.
Colour: similar to that of a pearl.
Surface: ulcerated with telangiectasia.
Margin: slightly raised and rolled, well defined (Fig. 8.11).

Cystic
Lesion: papule or nodule.
Colour: pearly.
Surface: smooth lobulated and telangiectatic (Fig. 8.12).

Morphoeic
Lesion: plaque.
Colour: pearly.
Surface: sclerodermatous (morphoeic) or scar-like with telangiectasia.

Pigmented
Any of those of the other types with the addition of visible pigment (Fig. 8.13).

Superficial
Lesion: plaque well defined.
Colour: red.
Surface: some scale.
Margin: fine rolled and pearly (Fig. 8.14).

Associations
- X-irradiation
  —and ankylosing spondylitis
  —and tinea capitis
- naevus sebaceous
- Gorlin–Goltz syndrome
- previous arsenic ingestion

Diagnosis
- histopathology (Fig. 8.15)
- cytology

Differential diagnosis
Of rodent ulcer, cystic, morphoeic and pigmented types:
- squamous cell carcinoma
- keratoacanthoma

Of the superficial basal cell carcinoma:
- Bowen's disease
- eczema
- psoriasis

Management
- surgical
- radiotherapy
- Mohs' chemosurgery
- topical 5-fluorouracil

Keratoacanthoma

Definition
A rapidly growing benign tumour, which simulates a squamous cell carcinoma but which involutes spontaneously within 4 months.

Characteristics

Symptoms
A spot which grows in an alarmingly rapid manner.

Signs
Lesion: a well-defined indurated papule which quickly becomes a discrete circumscribed nodule.
Colour: red.
Surface: has a central keratin-filled crater (Fig. 8.16).
Shape: dome shaped.
Margin: almost at an angle of 90° to the skin surface.

Distribution
Sun-damaged skin.

Special features
It involutes spontaneously after 4 months leaving behind a pitted scar.

Diagnosis
Histopathology.

Differential diagnosis
Squamous cell carcinoma.

Treatment
Surgical (either excision or curettage and cautery).

Malignant melanoma

Definition
An uncommon malignancy of melanocytes probably resulting from solar irradiation of Caucasian skin which may metastasize via lymphatics and the circulation.

Characteristics

Symptoms
Changes in behaviour of a pigmented lesion, which has either been present for many years or has recently been noticed by the patient. The suspicious changes are:

- increased growth (Fig. 8.17)
- changes in colour, particularly darkening (Fig. 8.19)
- changes in shape

Signs
Radial (horizontal) growth phase lesions:
- greater than 0.5 cm in size
- uneven distribution of shades and colours
- multiplicity of shades and colours
- irregular outline (scalloped) or notching (Fig. 8.20)
- subsequent very dark (usually black) local papule, nodule or plaque formation

Vertical (invasive) growth phase lesions:
- very dark (usually black) papule or nodule formation

Distribution
Anywhere but especially:
- lower limb (females)
- torso particularly back (males)
- face (elderly)

Progression
The lesion may metastasize particularly if the depth of invasion (Breslow thickness) is greater than 1.5 mm. Regional lymph nodes are usually involved first and then anywhere including lung, brain, liver and skin.

Variants
- amelanotic melanoma
- subungual (nail) melanoma

Diagnosis
- excision biopsy and histopathology
- Breslow thickness
- Clark's level (Table 8.2)

Classification

A. Horizontal growth phase lesions with subsequent vertical invasion

i. Hutchinson's lentigo maligna (melanoma):
- a disorder of the elderly
- usually on the face, neck or ear
- very slow horizontal growth phase
- ultimately may invade vertically causing tumour formation
- other signs of chronic sun damage
- easily visible but dismissed as an age spot and diagnosed late

Table 8.2 Clark's levels. This is the depth of invasion of the tumour defined by the anatomical site of the deepest tumour cell. Levels 4 and 5 are associated with a guarded prognosis

Level	Depth of infiltration of the dermis
1	Continued to the epidermis (*in situ*)
2	Infiltration of the papillary dermis
3	Infiltration to the junction of the papillary with the reticular dermis
4	Infiltration of the reticular dermis
5	Infiltration of the subcutaneous fat

Differential diagnosis
- solar lentigo
- seborrhoeic wart

ii. Superficial spreading malignant melanoma:
- initial horizontal growth phase (*in situ* melanoma)
- irregular outline (Fig. 8.18)
- irregular distribution of colours and pigment
- several different shades of colour and pigment
- subsequent vertical invasion and papule and nodule formation
- younger adults especially females
  Differential diagnosis
  - congenital melanocytic naevus
  - junctional naevus
  - compound naevus
  - dysplastic naevus
  - basal cell papilloma
  - solar lentigo
  - pigmented basal cell carcinoma

iii. Acral lentiginous (palmar plantar mucosal) malignant melanoma:
- irregular flat dark patch of pigmentation
- irregular outline
- early development of papular and nodular change
- palms, soles, mucosae
- most common in Orientals and Negroes
  Differential diagnosis
  - congenital naevus
  - junctional naevus
  - compound naevus
  - dysplastic naevus
  - melanotic freckle of the lip
  - trauma (black heel or 'talon noir')

B. Vertical invasion lesions *ab initio*

i. Papular (or nodular) malignant melanoma:
- predominantly black (Fig. 8.20)
- regular outline but often with a thin eccentric brown margin
- a nodule may bleed, ulcerate or lose pigment
  Differential diagnosis
  - haemangioma
  - dermatofibroma
  - blue naevus
  - compound naevus
  - dermal naevus
  - Spitz naevus
  - Reed's spindle cell tumour
  - angiokeratoma
  - neurofibroma

C. Special variants

i. Subungual melanoma:
- any nail
- grey or black discoloration under nail
- abnormal growth of nail, becoming distorted and split
- discoloration of skin around the nail, particularly at the nail fold (Hutchinson's sign)
  Differential diagnosis
  - haemorrhage under the nail secondary to trauma
  - *Pseudomonas* infection of the nail
  - linear melanonychia
  - fungus infection
  - subungual exostosis

ii. Amelanotic melanoma:
- a nodule
- commonly red and therefore mistaken for a haemangioma
- usually a tell-tale rim of pigment at the margin
  Differential diagnosis
  - haemangioma
  - pyogenic granuloma

Progression
- often initially to lymph nodes
- locally in transit metastases to the skin
- haematogenous spread to brain, lungs, liver, bones and elsewhere, including anywhere on the skin

Treatment
• surgical—wide excision (1 cm margin for each estimated 1 mm of invasion). May require reconstruction or skin grafting
• radiotherapy—sometimes for Hutchinson's lentigo on the face
• observation with serial photographs occasionally for Hutchinson's lentigo in the elderly and debilitated
• chemotherapy for metastatic disease

Prognosis (5-year survival)
Metastasis and survival is directly related to the depth of invasion of the tumour. The outcome in patients with thin lesions is usually good but the prognosis is more guarded in those with thick tumours. See Table 8.3.

Table 8.3 Five-year survival related to Breslow thickness

Breslow thickness (mm)	5-year survival rate (%)
<1.5	93
1.5–3.5	67
>3.5	37

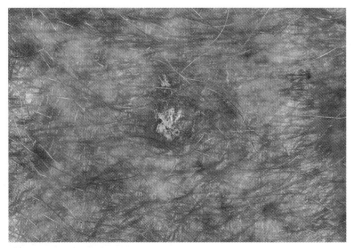

Fig. 8.1 Solar keratosis
The surface has a thick white adherent scale. A small percentage of keratoses increase in size and thickness and ultimately may become squamous cell carcinomas. Liquid nitrogen therapy is commonly employed but in this case curettage or excision would be most effective. It also provides material for histopathological examination.

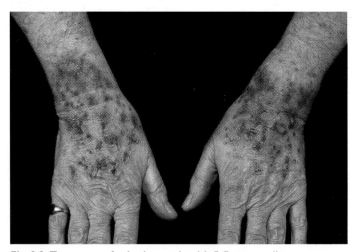

Fig. 8.2 Treatment of solar keratosis with 5-fluorouracil
Although cryotherapy is the standard treatment for solar keratoses they may recur and for multiple lesions 5-fluorouracil applied twice daily for 4 weeks is often very effective. The disadvantage is the inflammatory reaction which develops 10 days after treatment is begun. This patient was treated with a combination of 5-fluorouracil and retin A.

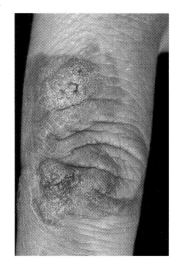

Fig. 8.3 Bowen's disease
There is a well-defined red plaque
on the back of the finger which is
part scaly and part hyperkeratotic. It
was mistaken for a long time for a
patch of eczema until a biopsy was
performed.

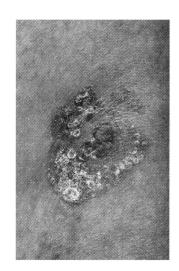

Fig. 8.4 Bowen's disease
The plaque could easily be mistaken
for psoriasis, although in the latter
disorder the scale is easily detached.
Also Bowen's disease is usually solitary and unilateral, whereas psoriasis is normally symmetrical.

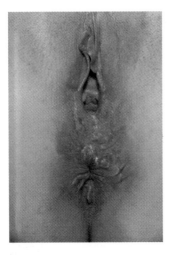

Fig. 8.5 Perianal and perivulval squamous cell carcinoma arising in Bowen's disease
There is a well-defined red–brown warty plaque around the anus and vulva which represents Bowen's disease. The lesion had been ignored and there is a nodular area posterior to the vulva which represents invasion into the dermis and thus squamous cell carcinoma.

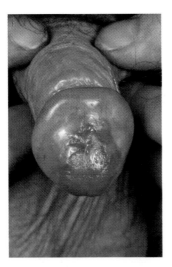

Fig. 8.6 Genital Bowen's disease progressing to squamous cell carcinoma
There is a well-defined red plaque on the glans penis with a small central papule. Biopsy is mandatory. The histopathology of the plaque showed intraepidermal carcinoma, but of the thicker papular area early squamous cell carcinoma. Topical 5-fluorouracil is not effective for squamous cell carcinoma and therefore surgery is indicated.

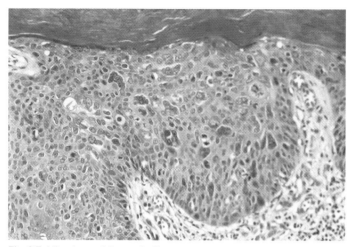

Fig. 8.7 Histology of Bowen's disease
This shows complete disorganization of the architecture of the epidermis with thickening and loss of polarity of the epithelial cells which are large and darkly staining and show numerous mitoses.

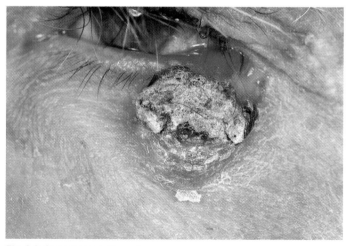

Fig. 8.8 Squamous cell carcinoma
As the lesion progresses, the thickening of the plaque becomes more apparent and crusting and ulceration become evident as a result of the disordered production of the epithelium. Note the ectropion resulting from retraction of the eyelid by the tumour.

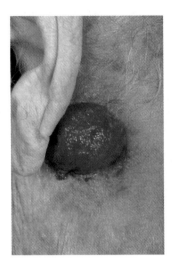

Fig. 8.9 Squamous cell carcinoma
This larger nodule has a raw eroded surface. The prognosis is guarded because of its size (lesions greater than 2 cm in diameter do not do well) and site. Lesions on and around the ear metastasize early.

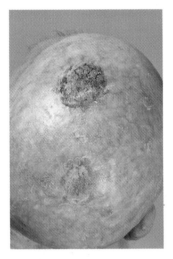

Fig. 8.10 Radiodermatitis secondary to treatment of scalp ringworm
Prior to the advent of oral griseofulvin in 1959, childhood scalp ringworm was treated with X-irradiation in order to cause epilation of the affected hairs. Over-irradiation resulted in atrophy, scarring, telangiectasia and pigmentation (radiodermatitis) which is clearly seen here and may result in skin cancer many decades later. Two crusted squamous cell carcinomas are visible. Similarly ultraviolet light frequently damages the prematurely bald scalp.

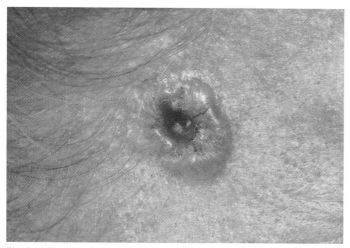

Fig. 8.11 Basal cell carcinoma
The most useful physical sign is the margin of the lesion. It has a pearly colour, is rolled and the surface is traversed by fine blood vessels (telangiectasia). Centrally there is ulceration. This is the classic rodent ulcer. The patient observes that it is a sore which tends to bleed, scab and fail to heal.

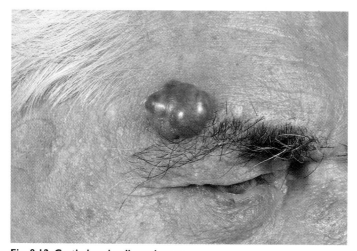

Fig. 8.12 Cystic basal cell carcinoma
This nodule has a lobulated smooth surface. Telangiectasia is evident with general erythema. There is no ulceration and these cystic lesions often attain a large size before diagnosis.

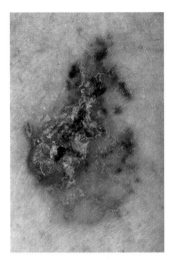

Fig. 8.13 Pigmented basal cell carcinoma
Sometimes the margin or even more of the lesion is pigmented which causes diagnostic confusion. Indeed the lesion may be mistaken for a superficial spreading melanoma. This is a superficial basal cell carcinoma which has become nodular and slightly ulcerated in the middle of the left-hand side.

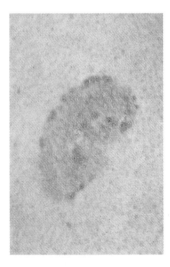

Fig. 8.14 Superficial basal cell carcinoma
Although frequently mistaken for a plaque of psoriasis or eczema it is usually solitary and certainly does not respond to topical steroids. The thin rolled outline to the lesion suggests the diagnosis and distinguishes it from Bowen's disease.

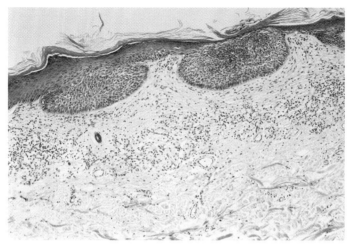

Fig. 8.15 Histopathology of superficial basal cell carcinoma
The basal cells bud down from the epidermis into the superficial dermis
and consequently are shallow enough to be reached and therefore
treated by topical 5-flourouracil.

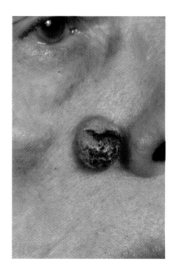

Fig. 8.16 Keratoacanthoma
The onset is sudden and growth
much swifter than in a squamous
cell carcinoma. The keratoacanthoma arises more abruptly from
the skin and has a pronounced
keratin-filled centre. Its resolution
probably represents the result of
immunosurveillance and rejection.
Squamous cell carcinomas are much
more common in the immunosuppressed, particularly transplant
recipients. Indeed the squamous cell
to basal cell ratio is reversed from
0.25:1 in normal individuals to 3:1
in the immunocompromised.

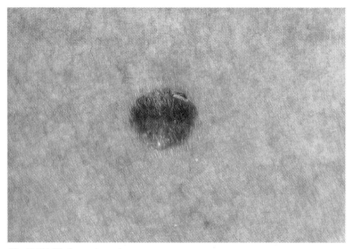

Fig. 8.17 Malignant melanoma
The commonest observation made by a patient with malignant melanoma is of increased growth of a 'mole' (pigmented lesion) as in this nodular melanoma.

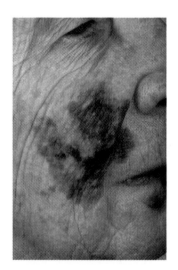

Fig. 8.18 Malignant melanoma
The face is the commonest site in the elderly. Lesions often grow to large proportions because in this age group the lesion is not recognized for what it is.

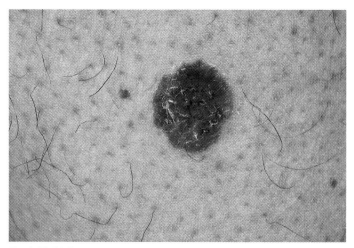

Fig. 8.19 Malignant melanoma
This 'mole' had been present all the patient's life but he had recently noticed a change in colour, and in particular darkening of the lesion.

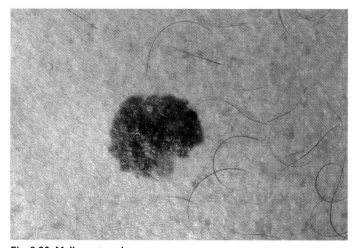

Fig. 8.20 Malignant melanoma
This superficial spreading malignant melanoma has an irregular content of pigment and had changed in shape producing a scalloped margin.

9 Bacterial Infections

Impetigo

Definition
An acute, contagious, rapidly spreading cutaneous infection due to either *Staphylococcus aureus* or a β-haemolytic *Streptococcus* or both, which commences as superficial purulent blisters which form golden crusts as they break, particularly affecting children and young people.

Characteristics

Symptoms
Blisters—acute onset, spreading.

Signs
Lesions:
• transient bullae containing purulent material
• fluid level may be discernible
• blisters break easily forming golden crusts; new lesions develop (Fig. 9.1)

Distribution
Anywhere, especially the face.

Variants
• sycosis barbae
• staphylococcal scalded skin syndrome (Lyell's disease) (Fig. 9.2)
• ecthyma (Fig. 9.3)

Diagnosis
• clinical
• investigation—swab for culture and sensitivity

Differential diagnosis
• insect bites—bullous types
• herpes simplex
• infected (impetiginized) eczema (Fig. 9.4)
• other blistering disorders

Management
Appropriate antibodies (usually flucloxacillin).

Folliculitis (Bockhart's impetigo)

Definition
An acute pustular eruption of hair follicles, caused by either *Staphylococcus aureus* or β-haemolytic streptococci or both, often associated with eczema or the treatment of inflammatory skin disorders with topical steroids.

Characteristics

Symptoms
Painful pus spots.

Signs
Lesions: pustules.
Colour: yellow or cream-coloured with surrounding erythema (Fig. 9.5).
Surface: hair in the centre of the pustule.
Shape: round.

Distribution
Anywhere, especially limbs.

Diagnosis
• clinical
• swab for culture and sensitivity including from carrier sites

Associations
Use of potent topical steroids, especially for psoriasis and eczema.

Differential diagnosis
• infected eczema
• acneiform folliculitis and ingrowing hairs
• HIV-associated eosinophilic folliculitis
• *Pseudomonas* folliculitis

Treatment
Antibiotics.

Furunculosis

Definition
An acute painful infection of the hair follicles which spreads into the surrounding dermis due to *Staphylococcus aureus*, which may be recurrent if associated with carriage of the bacterium in the nose or elsewhere.

Characteristics

Symptoms
Painful red lumps or 'boils'.

Signs
Lesions: oedematous red nodules with surrounding inflammation, often with a central yellow pustule and desquamation from the tension of the oedema.

Distribution
Anywhere but quite often near relevant *Staphylococcus aureus* carrier sites.

Diagnosis
- clinical
- swab of lesion and carrier sites for culture and sensitivities

Associations
Rarely diabetes mellitus.

Differential diagnosis
- acne conglobata
- hidradenitis suppurativa

Treatment
- systemic antibiotics
- local antibiotics for affected carrier sites
- occasionally incision and drainage

Erysipelas and cellulitis

Definition
An acute, sometimes recurrent, infection of the dermis and the upper (erysipelas) and entire (cellulitis) subcutaneous tissue of a leg or the face usually caused by *Streptococcus pyogenes* resulting in a high fever, rigors, vomiting and confusion.

Characteristics

Symptoms
Sudden illness, fever, hot painful red swollen face or limb.

Signs
Lesions: diffuse red, hot, oedematous, sometimes with surface pustules or vesicles (Fig. 9.6).

Distribution
- unilateral usually
- face or limb

Variants
Surgical erysipelas.

Diagnosis
- clinical
- swab any purulent material for culture and sensitivity

Associations
Occasionally:
- alcoholism
- malnourishment
- dysgammaglobulinaemia

Probably underlying lymphatic hypoplasia.
Sometimes tinea pedis or otitis externa (portal of entry).

Differential diagnosis
Facial erysipelas:
- herpes zoster
- contact dermatitis

Leg cellulitis:
- contact dermatitis

Surgical erysipelas:
- herpes zoster

Treatment
- systemic antibiotics
- long-term low-dose penicillin for recurrent attacks

Streptococcal toxic erythema

Definition
An acute widespread erythematous exanthem following after a group A β-haemolytic streptococcal throat infection which resolves after 7 days with desquamation particularly of the lips, palms and soles, and is a benign variant of scarlet fever.

Characteristics

Symptoms
A rash following a sore throat and fever.

Signs
Widespread blotchy erythema resolves by desquamation particularly of the lips, palms and soles (Fig. 9.7).

Distribution
Widespread and including palms and soles.

Associations
Preceding fever, sore throat and regional adenitis.

Diagnosis
- clinical
- raised white count with pronounced neutrophilia, sometimes eosinophilia
- throat swab for culture and sensitivity (and sometimes blood culture)
- antistreptolysin (ASO) titre

Differential diagnosis
- Kawasaki disease
- staphylococcal scalded skin syndrome
- of viral exanthems

Management
Penicillin V or erythromycin.

Erythrasma

Definition
An infection, caused by *Corynebacterium minutissimum*, of the warm, potentially damp, occluded areas of the skin such as the groin, axillae and under the breasts, producing a brown discoloration of the skin. Toe webs may also be infected but here the infection is clinically indistinguishable from tinea.

Characteristics

Symptoms
Asymptomatic, occasionally itchy, brown discoloration.

Signs
Lesions: a patch.
Colour: brown.
Surface: wrinkled with a fine scale (Fig. 9.8).
Shape: oval or round, well defined.

Distribution
- flexures
- axillae
- groins
- under pendulous breasts

Diagnosis
- clinical
- Wood's light examination—fluoresces coral-pink colour
- scrapings of skin for direct microscopy

Differential diagnosis
Other eruptions in the flexures.

Associations
- sometimes obesity
- hot humid environment

Treatment
- topical imidazoles or sodium fusidate
- oral erythromycin

Gonococcaemia

Definition
A dissemination of *Neisseria gonococcus*, which may occur if the primary stage of genitourinary or anal discharge has not been treated, resulting in fever, arthritis and an acral papulovesicular eruption, usually in females.

Characteristics

Symptoms
Malaise, fever, mono- or oligoarthritis and rash.

Signs
Lesions: scattered papulovesicles with a necrotic centre (Fig. 9.9).

Distribution
Extremities—fingers, palms, toes and soles.

Diagnosis
- clinical
- swabs from anus, urethra and vagina for culture and sensitivity

Differential diagnosis
Erythema multiforme (target lesions).

99

Treatment
Penicillin.

Meningococcaemia

Definition
An acute feverish illness resulting in meningitis, septicaemia and a purpuric rash due to *Neisseria meningitidis*.

Characteristics

Symptoms
Malaise, fever, headache, photophobia, neck stiffness, vomiting and a rash.

Signs
Lesions: several or many scattered purpuric macules (Fig. 9.10).

Distribution
Limbs and trunk.

Diagnosis
- clinical
- isolation of the Gram-positive diplococcus from the blood or cerebrospinal fluid

Differential diagnosis
Other purpuric eruptions.

Treatment
- penicillin (started as soon as the clinical diagnosis is made)
- chloramphenicol (in allergic subjects)

Syphilis

Definition
An infection with the spirochaete *Treponema pallidum*, usually sexually transmitted, resulting in a primary stage at the site of inoculation (chancre), a secondary systemic illness dominated by a rash and then, if untreated, resolution or resurgence with a tertiary stage particularly involving the cardiovascular and nervous systems.

PRIMARY STAGE (CHANCRE)

Characteristics

Symptoms
A painless sore occurring 9–90 days after infection, which heals without trace within 3 months.

Signs
A painless ulcer, with an indurated edge and firm base.

Distribution
- at the site of infection usually
- genitalia
- anus
- occasionally lip and finger

Diagnosis
Dark ground microscopic examination of base of chancre for treponemes.

Differential diagnosis
Other causes of anogenital ulcers.

SECONDARY STAGE

Characteristics

Symptoms
Malaise, fever, generalized enlargement of lymph nodes and an asymptomatic rash.

Signs
Lesions:
- pink macules (roseola)
- red–brown papules with a tendency to cropping (Fig. 9.11)
- firm red small plaques, often scaly, resembling psoriasis or pityriasis rosea
- may become annular
- may become moist and eroded in intertriginous areas

Distribution
Widespread but especially:
- palms and soles
- face
- genitalia
- mucous membranes (Fig. 9.12)
- the scalp, causing hair loss

Diagnosis
Positive serological tests.

Differential diagnosis
- guttate psoriasis
- pityriasis rosea

TERTIARY SYPHILIS

Gumma

Characteristics

Symptoms
A painless ulcer.

Signs
Lesions: a punched-out ulcer with a chamois-leather-like base: multiple gummata coalesce making geometrical or scalloped patterns.

Distribution
- scalp
- face
- palate
- legs

Nodular or tubercular syphilide

Characteristics

Symptoms
Asymptomatic plaque(s).

Signs
Lesions: papules or nodules.
Colour: copper-coloured.
Shape: circinate, kidney or horseshoe shaped.
Surface: scaly (psorasiform) or crusted.

Distribution
Anywhere but particularly face and extensor surfaces of limbs and back.

Late mucous membrane lesions

Characteristics

Symptoms
Tongue: glazed areas with loss of papillae leading to leukoplakia ulceration and scarring which in the palate may result in perforation.

Lyme disease

Definition
An infection caused by the spirochaete, *Borrelia burgdorferi*, transmitted by a tick infected from an animal reservoir, resulting in an annular erythema, which if not treated may have neurological and rheumatological consequences.

Characteristics

Symptoms
A red ring on the skin.

Signs
Lesions: an annular erythema spreading outwards with possibly a central papule from a tick bite (Fig. 9.13).

Distribution
Anywhere.

Diagnosis
• clinical
• ELISA assay for antigens (not always positive)

Differential diagnosis
• granuloma annulare
• other annular lesions

Complications
• Neurological: a triad of cranial polyneuropathy, a painful radiculopathy and chronic meningitis
• myocarditis
• polyarthralgia and sometimes a chronic asymmetrical oligoarthritis

Management
Oral tetracycline or penicillin.

Leprosy

Definition

A tropical infection transmitted by nasal droplets infected with *Mycobacterium leprae,* which invade the Schwann cells and involve primarily the skin and nervous system to a degree depending on the immunological status of the patient and the bacterial load. The disease is thus classified as a spectrum which ranges from tuberculoid via borderline to lepromatous types.

TUBERCULOID LEPROSY

Characteristics

Symptoms
One or several anaesthetic ringed patches on the skin, thickened peripheral nerves, and palsies.

Signs
Lesions: patch(es).
Colour: hypopigmented or red with central hypopigmentation (Fig. 9.14).
Surface: dry, scaly, does not sweat, anaesthetic.
Shape: annular.

Distribution
Cool peripheral areas of the body especially:
• buttocks
• elbows
• knees
• extensor surfaces of limbs and face

Complications
Involvement of peripheral nerves especially ulnar, peroneal and great auricular, resulting in peripheral neuropathy with sensory changes and palsies, e.g. foot or wrist drop.

LEPROMATOUS LEPROSY

Characteristics

Symptoms
Widespread rash.

Signs
Lesions: multiple symmetrical macules or patches which gradually become infiltrated and nodular.

Distribution
Widespread, with sparing of scalp, axillae, groin and perineum, with a tendency to nodule formation on the nose, ears (Fig. 9.15), lips and forehead.

Complications
• sensory and motor changes
• ocular, nasal, testicular, renal and other system involvement
• reversal reactions (oedema of skin lesions and nerves resulting in acute damage)
• erythema nodosum leprosum (immune complete reaction)

Diagnosis
• smears for slit-skin samples
• histopathology

Differential diagnosis
• other annular lesions
• hypopigmented lesions
• nodular lesions

Management
• complicated
• referral to a leprologist for multidrug regiment including rifampicin, clofazimine and dapsone

Tuberculosis

Definition
An infection caused by *Mycobacterium tuberculosis* which may invade the skin directly from a focus in a bone, joint or lymph node (lupus vulgaris) or from direct inoculation (including Bacillus Calmette–Guérin (BCG) vaccination). It quite commonly results in an immune complex disorder (erythema induratum). Occasionally atypical species may invade the skin, for example *Mycobacterium balnei* in people who keep fish and *Mycobacterium avium* in patients with HIV disease.

Characteristics (lupus vulgaris)

Symptoms
A solitary symptomless patch (Fig. 9.16).

Signs
Lesions: a plaque.
Colour: red–brown.
Shape: well-defined irregular outline.
Surface: may be scaly and atrophic.

Distribution
Usually either face or limb.

Diagnosis
Skin biopsy shows a granulomatous infiltrate.

Differential diagnosis
- Bowen's disease
- lupus erythematosus
- tertiary syphilis

Associations of tuberculosis
- erythema induratum
- atypical mycobacteria

Management
- prevention with BCG vaccination
- antituberculous therapy

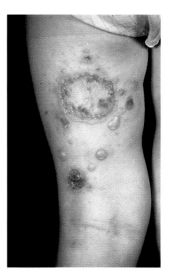

Fig. 9.1 Impetigo
The blisters may attain quite a large size. As they break, yellow–brown crusts form. It is a common disorder of childhood. The diagnosis is made clinically but the relevant organism may be determined by taking a swab for culture and sensitivity. A *Staphylococcus* is usually penicillin resistant.

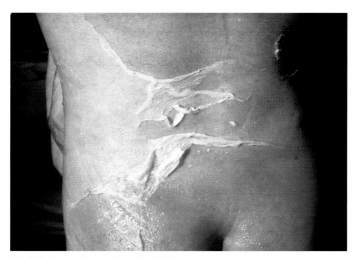

Fig. 9.2 Staphylococcal scalded skin syndrome
This is due to an epidermolytic exotoxin from a group 2 staphylococcus (phage-type 71). It is uncommon. The child is ill, crying (because the skin is burning and tender to touch) and feverish. There is redness and peeling of the epidermis into sheets, leaving raw denuded skin beneath. Early recognition and treatment may be life-saving.

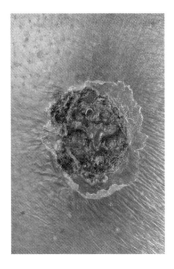

Fig. 9.3 Ecthyma
This is a deeper bacterial infection than impetigo. The purulent material forms yellow–brown crusts, surrounded by erythema and desquamation of the skin secondary to the oedema, with erosions underneath. It is common in tropical climates.

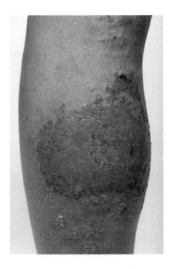

Fig. 9.4 Infected eczema
There is an oozing, raw and purulent area often surrounded by dry pink scaly patches of atopic eczema. Eczema often becomes secondarily infected but does not respond to antibiotics alone. Topical steroids are also required.

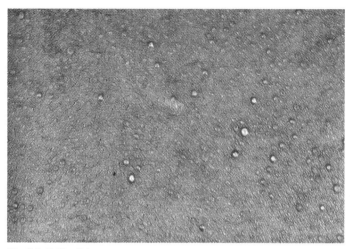

Fig. 9.5 Folliculitis
There are cream- or yellow-coloured pustules surrounding a hair shaft.
The most common cause is the bacterium, *Staphylococcus aureus*. It may
occur as a primary infection or as a complication in patients with
eczema or psoriasis who have been using potent or superpotent topical
steroids too generously.

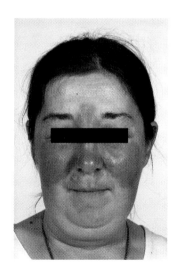

Fig. 9.6 Erysipelas
Often unilateral, sometimes bilateral, the skin is hot, bright red and
oedematous. The patient is unwell,
feverish, may vomit and become
delerious. The onset is abrupt.

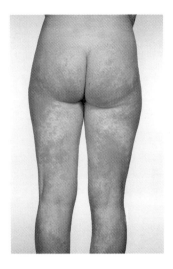

Fig. 9.7 Streptococcal toxic erythema
This young woman had a severe sore throat with enlarged tonsils, regional adenitis and fever followed shortly afterwards by a widespread blotchy erythema with involvement of the palms and soles, with subsequent desquamation. A Group A β-haemolytic streptococcus was isolated from a throat swab. This is the common form of scarlet fever which is otherwise rarely seen in the West. Penicillin is the treatment of choice.

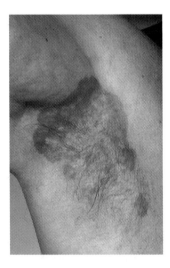

Fig. 9.8 Erythrasma
This is an infection of intertriginous sites by *Corynebacterium minutissimum*. The axillae or groin are affected by a brown discolouration of the skin with a fine scaly wrinkled surface. It responds to topical sodium fusidate or imidazoles. Oral erythromycin is equally effective.

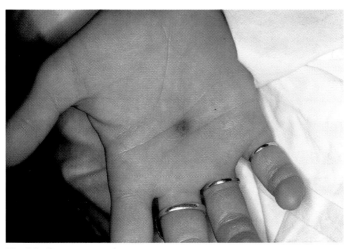

Fig. 9.9 Gonococcaemia
Gonorrhoea is usually diagnosed in its earliest stages with a urethral, vaginal or anal discharge. However, in females in particular, this may be minimal and gonococcaemia supervenes. The patient is feverish and has an arthritis affecting one or several joints asymmetrically with sparse discreet haemorrhagic vesiculopustules on the extremities especially palms, fingers, soles and toes. © Photograph courtesy of Dr Frank Dann, Los Angeles.

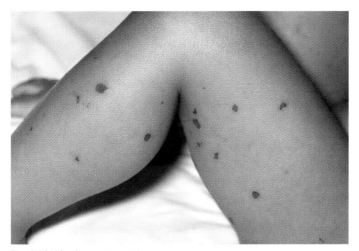

Fig. 9.10 Meningococcaemia
This is an acute, potentially lethal, meningitis with septicaemia caused by a Gram-positive diplococcus. There are small purpuric papules due to direct invasion of the cutaneous blood vessels by *Neisseria meningitidis*. High-dose penicillin or chloramphenicol should be given immediately the diagnosis is suspected.

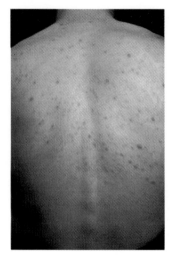

Fig. 9.11 Secondary syphilis
If the chancre is untreated, a secondary systemic stage of malaise, fever, generalized lymphadenopathy and widespread rash ensues. It is initially macular and pink (roseola), then papular, becoming a copper colour and ultimately more infiltrated and annular. It is characteristically nonpruritic.

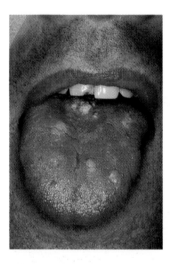

Fig. 9.12 Secondary syphilis
There are grey–white patches scattered over the dorsal surface of the tongue; these are characteristic of the secondary stage of the disease.

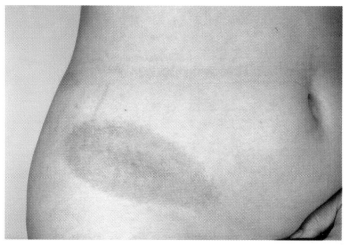

Fig. 9.13 Lyme disease
This disease is caused by *Borrelia burgdorferi,* a spirochaete which is transmitted by infected ticks. The patient is bitten by a tick and the infection results in a red ring spreading outwards from the original site of the bite.

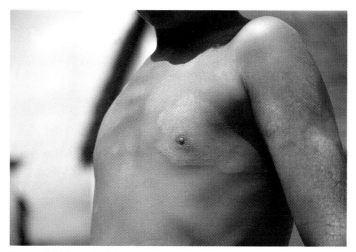

Fig. 9.14 Tuberculoid leprosy
There are hypopigmented annular patches which are anaesthetic to pinprick and light touch. The surface is dry (the area does not sweat) and slightly scaly. There is high immunological resistance to *M. leprae* which results in peripheral nerve thickening and damage.

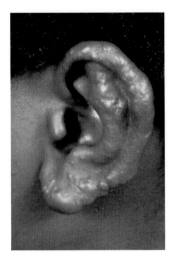

Fig. 9.15 Lepromatous leprosy
Papules and nodules are widespread
and fairly symmetrical. This form of
the disease is contagious from nasal
droplet infection. Antilepromatous
treatment renders it rapidly unin-
fectious. Ultimately diffuse infiltration results in deep fissuring of the
skin producing a somewhat leonine
appearance.

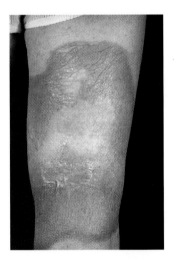

Fig. 9.16 Lupus vulgaris
There is a very well-defined
red–brown plaque on the upper leg.
The condition is very rare in the
West and is usually secondary to a
tuberculous focus in a bone, joint or
lymph node.

10 Fungal Infections

TINEA (RINGWORM)

An infection caused by a superficial fungus which colonizes keratin—that is hair, nails or the stratum corneum—but does not ordinarily penetrate into living cells. The fungus is a dermatophyte, a multicellular organism consisting of branching hyphae which mat together to form mycelia. It may originate from an animal (zoophilic), a human (anthropophilic) or occasionally a soil (geophilic) source.

Tinea capitis

Characteristics

Symptoms
Patchy loss of scalp hair in a child (Fig. 10.1).

Signs
Lesions:
- round patches of alopecia with red, purulent and inflamed skin, *or*
- slightly scaly and pink (minimal inflammation) depending on the species

Distribution
- scalp
- may have skin involvement (usually neck)

Special features
Kerion: a boggy mass of inflamed and purulent skin due to a vigorous host response to an animal fungus.
Favus: a scarring alopecia due to *Trichophyton schoenleinii*.

Diagnosis
- clinical
- microscopy of affected hairs and skin
- culture of this material
- microsporum species fluoresce a brilliant green under Wood's light

Associations
Radiodermatitis and skin cancer, a long-term consequence of treatment of scalp ringworm with X-rays.

Differential diagnosis
- alopecia areata
- pityriasis amiantacea
- other disorders of the scalp

Treatment
- oral griseofulvin or terfenadine
- pulse itraconazole

Tinea corporis

Characteristics

Symptoms
A spreading itchy rash.

Signs
Lesions: patch(es).
Colour: red.
Surface: scaling at the margin (Fig. 10.2).
Shape: annular with a tendency to central healing and post-inflammatory pigmentation (Fig. 10.3).

Distribution
Asymmetrically on smooth skin.

Variants
- tinea facei
- tinea barbae
- tinea under the watch strap (Fig. 10.5)
- tinea incognito

Diagnosis
- clinical
- microscopy (Fig. 10.4)
- culture

Differential diagnosis
- discoid eczema
- granuloma annulare
- discoid psoriasis
- the herald patch of pityriasis rosea
- any annular eruption

Tinea cruris

Characteristics

Symptoms
An itchy rash in the groin.

Signs
Lesions: patches.
Colour: pink.
Surface: scaling at the periphery.
Shape: tendency to be arranged in annular patterns.

Distribution
• groin, advancing down inner thigh away from genitocrural folds (scrotum is rarely involved) (Fig. 10.6)
• may spread to the buttocks

Variants
Tinea incognito.

Associations
Tinea pedis and unguis.

Differential diagnosis
• erythrasma
• candidosis
• psoriasis
• seborrhoeic eczema
• lichen simplex
• lichen planus
• other disorders in the groin

Tinea pedis

Characteristics

Symptoms
Itching and scaling of the feet and between the toes ('athlete's foot').

Signs
Acute:
• vesicles and bullae usually on one sole of the foot
Chronic:
• crescentic scaling of soles and webs of toes
• white powdery filling-in of skin creases

Variants

Tinea incognito.

Associations

Tinea of the nails.

Diagnosis

- clinical
- microscopy
- culture

Differential diagnosis

Of acute tinea:
- podopompholyx
- pustular psoriasis

Of chronic tinea:
- eczema
- psoriasis

Of toe web tinea:
- pseudomonas
- soft corn

Of any foot eruption

Tinea manuum

Characteristics

Symptoms

A rash usually on one hand only, often with abnormal finger nails.

Signs

- dryness and scaling with some erythema
- white, powdery skin creases (Fig. 10.7)
- usually involvement of one or more finger nails

Distribution

One palm only.

Associations

Involvement of both soles of feet and toe nails.

Diagnosis

- clinical
- microscopy
- culture

Differential diagnosis
- *Scytalidium hyalinum* infection
- eczema
- psoriasis
- of any palmar eruption

Management of tinea

Local remedies
- half-strength Whitfield's ointment
- undecenoic acid
- tolnaftate
- imidazoles
- Castellani's paint with or without magenta—for acute tinea pedis
- potassium permanganate—for acute tinea pedis
- tioconazole (for nail infections)

Systemic therapy
- griseofulvin
- itraconazole
- terbinafine

Indications for systemic therapy of tinea
Absolute:
- tinea capitis
- tinea of the nails
- *Trichophyton rubrum* infection
Relative:
- tinea incognito

CANDIDA

An opportunistic infection with a yeast which is normally a commensal and which principally affects the mouth, genitalia, nail folds and intertriginous skin.

Oral candidosis (thrush)

Characteristics

Symptoms
Sore mouth.

Signs
Lesions: cream or whitish pustules which become confluent, raw and eroded.

Distribution
- palate
- tongue

Variants
Angular cheilitis.

Associations
- dentures and poor oral hygiene
- immunosuppression

Diagnosis
- clinical
- culture

Differential diagnosis
- lichen planus
- other oral disorders

Candida vulvovaginitis

Characteristics

Symptoms
Vaginal irritation, soreness and a thick creamy discharge.

Signs (cutaneous)
Lesions: pustules which coalesce and erode with redness and swelling (Fig. 10.8) and satellite pustules peripheral to the main site of the eruption.

Distribution
Around the vulva and may spread perianally and onto the inner thigh.

Associations
- pregnancy
- oral contraceptives
- antibiotics
- diabetes mellitus (especially older patients)

Diagnosis
- clinical
- swabs of lesions and vagina for microbiology

Differential diagnosis
Other vulval lesions.

Candida balanitis

Characteristics

Symptoms
A rash on the penis.

Signs
Cream-coloured pustules sometimes with swelling and erythema.

Distribution
Under prepuce on glans penis.

Diagnosis
- clinical
- swab for microbiology

Differential diagnosis
Other penile lesions.

Candida intertrigo

Characteristics

Symptoms
Rash in the flexures, particularly groin (or napkin area) or under the breasts.

Signs
Lesions: small cream-coloured pustules on an erythematous base which coalesce and erode and are often surrounded by maceration.

Distribution
- groin, sometimes axillae
- sub-mammary

Variants
- erosio interdigitale
- candida paronychia (Fig. 16.10)

Diagnosis
Swab for microbiology.

Differential diagnosis
Other flexural eruptions.

Management of candidosis

- local imidazoles or nystatin (including suspensions, lozenges, pessaries and creams)
- systemic imidazoles and triazoles
- treatment of underlying cause

PITYRIASIS VERSICOLOR

Definition

An infection occurring mainly after puberty caused by a unicellular yeast *Pityrosporum ovale* or *orbiculare* which is normally present on the trunk as a commensal. It produces brown-coloured and hypopigmented macules on the torso.

Characteristics

Symptoms

A rash on the body which often disturbs the pigment of the skin (versicolor).

Signs

Lesions: macules which become confluent.
Colour: fawn coloured (Fig. 10.9) or off white (Fig. 10.10).
Surface: slight fine scale (pityriasis) often only visible if the lesion is scraped with a blunt scalpel.
Shape: well-defined polymorphic.

Distribution

- asymmetrical
- back and front of chest
- abdomen and upper limbs in more extensive infections
- rarely face

Special features

Pseudovitiligo.

Diagnosis

- clinical
- direct microscopy

Associations

Immunosuppression.

Causes

- solar irradiation
- AIDS

- lymphoma
- Cushing's disease
- systemic steroids
- topical steroids

Differential diagnosis

- pityriasis rosea
- vitiligo

Management

- topical imidazoles
- oral triazoles

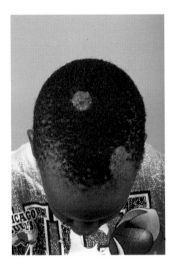

Fig. 10.1 Tinea capitis

Tinea capitis affects children and the striking physical sign is a round area of hair loss. This becomes inflamed and scaly. The diagnosis may be confirmed by examining skin scales and hair under the microscope for the presence of spores and hyphae. Treatment is with oral griseofulvin for at least 6 weeks although this will be superseded by oral terfenadine.

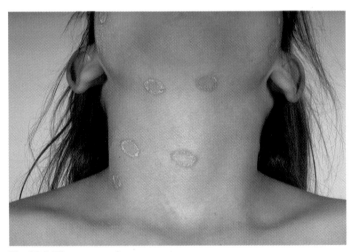

Fig. 10.2 Tinea corporis

This is the clinical appearance known as ringworm. The lesions are annular, being more pronounced peripherally and with a tendency to central clearing. This may spread in a child from the scalp (usually *Trichophyton tonsurans*) or be due to direct infection usually from a puppy or kitten (*Microsporum canis*).

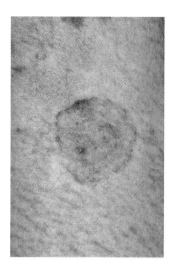

Fig. 10.3 Tinea corporis
This is ringworm, a red ring-shaped patch with a more pronounced scaling margin and a tendency to central clearing and hyperpigmentation.

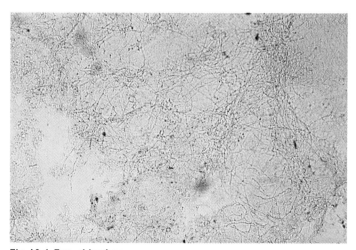

Fig. 10.4 Fungal hyphae
Branching filaments, known as hyphae, are present. Scrapings can be taken from the skin with a blunt scalpel. The scales are put onto a glass slide and potassium hydroxide is added to dissolve the keratin and reveal the hyphae crossing over the epidermal cell walls.

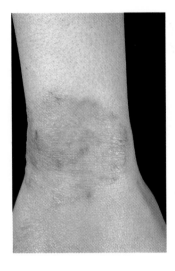

Fig. 10.5 Tinea corporis
The occlusive conditions of slight moisture and warmth provided by a watch and its strap favour the growth of tinea, particularly *Trichophyton rubrum* spreading from the feet. The diagnosis of eczema is usually made and the patient is prescribed topical steroids which permit the fungus to flourish even more. Note the scaling at the margin.

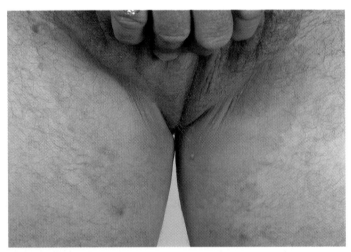

Fig. 10.6 Tinea cruris
This itchy eruption does not usually involve the scrotum but moves down the inner upper thigh away from the genitocrural fold. It is red and scaly, particularly at the periphery of the rash.

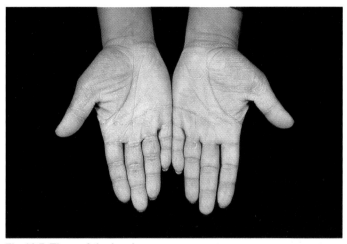

Fig. 10.7 Tinea of the hand
Tinea usually only affects the skin and fingernails of one hand, although both feet are involved. It is due to *Trichophyton rubrum*. There is a fine powder-like scale, particularly in the skin creases.

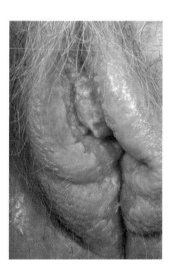

Fig. 10.8 Candida vulvovaginitis
There is oedema of the vulva, with maceration due to coalescence of the pustules which are the initial lesions in candidosis, which subsequently result in raw erosions. This octogenarian woman was found to have glycosuria. Candida vulvovaginitis is a common presentation of diabetes mellitus.

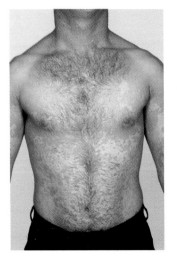

Fig. 10.9 Pityriasis versicolor
There is extensive involvement with fawn-coloured macules with a slight scale. Although it is a common disorder due to the commensal *P. ovale* or *P. orbiculare* often precipitated by the warmth and sweat induced by the sun, it also occurs in the immunosuppressed, such as those with lymphoma, Cushing's and AIDS. Misdiagnosis and treatment with topical steroids is the commonest immunosuppressive cause.

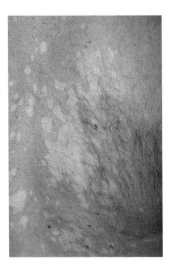

Fig. 10.10 Pityriasis versicolor
In a suntanned individual the affected skin looks pale and hypopigmented. The 'change' in colour gives rise to its name of versicolor. The fungus produces a dicarboxylic acid which temporarily interferes with melanin production from the melanocytes. After treatment it takes several months to recover.

11 Viral Infections

Herpes simplex

Definition
An acute contagious short-lived (7–12 days) infection of the skin or mucous membranes caused by a double-stranded DNA virus, herpes virus hominis, which results in a primary attack (often subclinical) with subsequent less marked recurrences, principally precipitated by fever, stress, menstruation or ultraviolet irradiation.

Characteristics

Symptoms
A 'cold' sore: premonitory symptoms of itch or tingling.

Signs
Lesions: initially macules which progress as vesicles surrounded by erythema to vesiculopustules and then crusts before healing sometimes with post-inflammatory pigmentation (Fig. 11.1).
Configuration: grouped.

Distribution
Anywhere but particularly on the cheeks, in and around the mouth, fingers, buttocks and genitalia.

Variants and complications
• neonatal herpes simplex
• herpes simplex and erythema multiforme
• keratoconjunctivitis
• eczema herpeticum
• herpetic whitlow

Diagnosis
• clinical
• cytology (Tzank smear)
• electron microscopy
• culture

Differential diagnosis
Of facial lesions.
• impetigo
• herpes zoster
Of herpes stomatitis:

- Coxsackie infections
- other oral lesions

Of genital herpes simplex:
- Other genital lesions

Treatment
- prevention (avoid contact during an outbreak)
- topical acyclovir (minor recurrences)
- systemic acyclovir (primary attacks, neonatal infections, eczema herpeticum, frequent recurrences)

Varicella (chickenpox)

Definition
A common infection occurring in epidemics in young people caused by the varicella-zoster virus (VZV), lasting 2 weeks, associated with a mild fever, malaise and a pruritic predominantly vesicular skin eruption.

Characteristics

Symptoms
A widespread rash following a day or two after a mild prodrome of fever and malaise.

Signs
Lesions: a rapid progression from red macules and papules which become vesicles with at first clear and subsequently turbid contents, surrounded by erythema, which in turn dry, crust and heal with minimal scarring. *Configuration*: appear in crops (Fig. 11.2).

Distribution
Centripetal and intraoral.

Complications
- neonatal chickenpox
- haemorrhagic chickenpox in the immunosuppressed
- keloid scars

Differential diagnosis
Other truncal eruptions presenting acutely.

Management
Rest and symptomatic therapy:
- acyclovir for patients at risk

Prevention of chickenpox:

• live attenuated virus (preventative in the healthy, modifies it in those at risk)
• specific immune globulin (reduces severity: indicated in the perinatal period if mother of the child has chickenpox: often given with acyclovir)

Herpes zoster (shingles)

Definition
A painful infection of cutaneous nerves with a double-stranded DNA virus belonging to the herpes group. It is a reactivation of the dormant virus of chickenpox and hence is known as the varicella zoster virus.

Characteristics

Symptoms
A painful rash and slight malaise.

Signs
Lesions: a rapid progression from red macules to vesicles surrounded by erythema which may become confluent. These become vesiculopustules haemorrhagic scabs and subsequently heal with scarring, particularly if secondarily infected with staphylococci.

Distribution
Unilateral corresponding to a dermatome (Fig. 11.3).

Complications
• ocular (involvement of the nasociliary ganglion of the ophthalmic branch of the trigeminal nerve)
• Ramsay Hunt syndrome (involvement of geniculate ganglion resulting in a facial palsy)
• retention of urine or faeces (involvement of sacral nerve)
• paralysis of the affected limb (usually temporary)
• disseminated herpes zoster
• post-herpetic neuralgia
• contagious to associates who have not had chickenpox

Diagnosis
• clinical
• tissue culture
• electron microscopy
• complement-fixing antibodies in acute and convalescent sera

Differential diagnosis
• erysipelas/cellulitis
• zonal herpes simplex

Management

Herpes zoster:
- acyclovir 800 mg five times daily for 1 week
- fanciclovir
- topical acyclovir
- adequate analgesia and rest

Ramsay Hunt syndrome:
- acyclovir with systemic steroids (to reduce inflammation)

Post-herpetic neuralgia:
- amitriptyline
- carbamazepine
- topical capsaicin 0.025%

Warts

Definition

A very common infection with a human papilloma virus (HPV), of which there are a large number of subtypes as determined by DNA hybridization, each of which may be associated with an affinity for particular anatomical sites or clinical appearance.

Characteristics

Common warts

Lesions: discrete papules which may become confluent forming plaques.
Colour: flesh-coloured or off-white.
Surface: roughened.
Distribution: anywhere especially hands, fingers, knees, face and around the nails.

Plane warts (Fig. 11.4)

Lesions: small papules, often in profusion.
Colour: flesh-coloured or pigmented.
Surface: flat topped, slightly roughened.
Distribution: face, backs of hands and shins. Koebner phenomenon (linear arrangement) may be present.

Plantar warts (verrucae)

Deep 'myrmecia' (Greek *myrmax*—having the configuration of an ant hill): sharply defined, rounded lesion with a rough warty surface surrounded by a collar of thickened horn.
Mosaic: lesion consisting of a plaque made up of individual papules compacted together, the margins of which are easily discernible.

Anogenital warts (condyloma acuminatum)

Lesions: papules often filiform, pedunculated, acuminate (= pointed) or papillomatous.
Colour: pink, soft.

Filiform or digitate warts

Distribution: mainly on the face.

Variants

• warts in immunosuppressed patients (Fig. 11.7)
• warts and oncogenicity

Differential diagnosis

Not usually a problem except:
Plane warts on face:
• acne
• other facial eruptions (especially papular)
Verrucae:
• corns
Genital warts:
• pearly penile papules
• other genital lesions

Management

• weak acids (gels, paints and plasters)
• cryotherapy
• curettage
• immunotherapy
• natural resolution

Molluscum contagiosum

Definition

A contagious cutaneous infection with a poxvirus which produces multiple dome-shaped papules with an umbilicated centre which occur over a number of months before disappearing spontaneously. It is more common in children, particularly atopics and in association with HIV infections.

Characteristics

Symptoms

An eruption of spots.

Signs

Lesions: papules.
Colour: flesh-coloured or red-brown.

Shape: hemispherical or dome shaped.
Surface: a central umbilication (Fig. 11.5).
Surrounding skin: may become inflamed or eczematous as the lesion involutes.

Variants
Occasionally solitary.

Associations
• more common in atopics
• HIV-infected patients are more susceptible

Diagnosis
• clinical
• curettage of a lesion for histopathology (Fig. 11.6)

Differential diagnosis
• warts
• intradermal naevus
• syringoma
• senile sebaceous hyperplasia
• milia
• naevoxanthoendothelioma

Management
Cryotherapy if required.

COMMON CHILDHOOD AND EPIDEMIC EXANTHEMS

Erythema subitum (roseola infantum)

Definition
The commonest exanthem under the age of 2 due to human herpes virus 6 (HHV-6), presenting abruptly (subitum) with a high fever of 4 days' duration which disappears with the arrival of the exanthem which lasts 2 days.

Characteristics

Symptoms
A high fever followed by a rash in infancy.

Signs
Discrete rose-pink maculopapules.

Distribution
Starts on the neck and trunk and progresses to the face and limbs.

Other features
Cervical and occipital lymphadenopathy.

Complications
Febrile convulsions without sequelae.

Diagnosis
- clinical
- human herpes virus 6 antibodies in blood

Differential diagnosis
Other febrile exanthems.

Management
Nil specific.

Hand, foot and mouth disease

Definition
A Coxsackie (usually A16) infection of young children but occasionally of institutionalized adults causing a mild stomatitis and vesicular eruption of the palms and soles lasting 7 days with little constitutional disturbance.

Characteristics

Symptoms
A rash on the hands and feet.

Signs
Oral white or pearly grey vesicles with a narrow red surround.

Distribution (Fig. 11.8)
- palms and soles
- around digits and nails
- in the mouth

Diagnosis
- clinical
- rarely inoculation into newborn mice or tissue culture of material from faeces, vesicles or nasopharynx

Differential diagnosis
Erythema multiforme.

Management
Symptomatic.

Erythema infectiosum (slapped cheek disease)

Definition

A sudden infection without prodrome caused by human parvovirus B19 producing a widespread exanthem with a characteristic erythema of the cheeks, lasting a few days but with a tendency to recur for 2–3 weeks in children and associated with a polyarthralgia in adults. It crosses the placenta and causes hydrops fetalis and intrauterine death in 10% of pregnancies.

Characteristics

Symptoms

A widespread rash but with cheeks which look as if they have been slapped.

Signs

Lesions: papules which coalesce to produce a blotchy, hot, turgid erythema especially on the cheeks ('slapped cheeks' appearance); macules and papules which form a lace-like patterning on the trunk and limbs.

Distribution

- widespread on trunk, limbs, hands and feet
- characteristic blotchiness on the cheeks (Fig. 11.9)
- may involve buccal and genital membranes with dark macules

Evolution

Lasts up to 10 days but may fade and recur in response to sunlight and heat over 3 or 4 weeks.

Complications

- polyarthritis in adults
- hydrops fetalis and intrauterine death if contracted during pregnancy in 10%

Diagnosis

- clinical
- IgM antibodies present for 2 months after infection
- electron microscopy of serum-virus discernible during acute phase

Differential diagnosis

See Table 11.1.

Treatment

None.

Table 11.1 The distinguishing features of the common epidemic febrile rashes

	Erythema subitum	Erythema infectiosum	Rubella	Measles
Prodrome	An infant with a high fever which resolves with sudden onset of rash on day 4	No	Not in children Brief in older	Yes Distinctive Lasts 3–5 days
Lymphadenopathy	Yes	No	Yes	No
Enanthem	No	Yes	20%	Koplick spots
Rash	Discrete rose-pink macules	'Slapped cheeks' Lace-like, maculopapular	Discrete pink macules become confluent and disappear in 24 hours	Day 4 Red macules becoming dull red blotches Desquamates
Distribution	Starts on neck and trunk; spreads to face and limbs	Cheeks Torso Limbs	Starts on face; spreads to trunk and limbs	Begins on forehead and behind ears; spreads everywhere
Duration	2 days	10 days (may recur)	4 days	6–10 days
Associations	Febrile convulsions	Polyarthritis (adults) Fetal damage	Polyarthritis (adults) Fetal damage	Bronchospasm Otitis media Encephalitis

German measles (rubella)

Definition
An epidemic infection of children and young adults caused by droplet infection from a togavirus resulting in an exanthem and lymphadenopathy, especially of the head and neck, sometimes complicated by an arthritis and serious fetal damage if contracted during pregnancy.

Characteristics

Symptoms
A rash without prodrome except in adults (fever, headache, malaise, sore throat and suffusion of the conjunctivae).

Signs
• discrete pink macules which become confluent and clear after 24 hours
• complete clearance by the 4th day

Distribution
Starts on the face, progresses to the trunk and then to the limbs.

Other features
Lymphadenopathy is present before the rash. It is general but especially involves the suboccipital, postauricular and cervical glands.

Complications
• arthritis (in adults especially females)
• congenital rubella syndrome, the main features of which are:
  —heart (especially patent ductus)
  —eye (especially cataract)
  —deafness
  —mental retardation and microcephaly
  —thrombocytopenia
  —jaundice
  —prematurity
  —spontaneous abortion
  —still birth

Diagnosis
• sequential serology
• IgM antibodies (positive at 14 days)

Differential diagnosis
See Table 11.1.

Management
• prophylaxis

- active immunization with MMR (measles, mumps and rubella) vaccination in second year of life
- no specific treatment

Measles

Definition
An epidemic infection caused by a paramyxovirus commencing with an acute prodrome of fever, malaise, catarrh, cough, conjunctivitis and photophobia accompanied by Koplick's spots followed on the 4th day by an exanthem which lasts about 10 days.

Characteristics

Symptoms
A rash following a fever and upper respiratory tract symptoms.

Signs
Red macules initially which become dull red blotchy papules which subsequently desquamate with some brown staining (Fig. 11.11).

Distribution
Starts on the forehead and behind the ears; spreads to the rest of the face, trunk and limbs.

Complications
Immediate:
- bronchopneumonia
- otitis media
- encephalitis
Delayed:
- subacute sclerosing panencephalitis
- tuberculosis

Diagnosis
Specific antibodies (present within 4 days of rash).

Differential diagnosis
See Table 11.1.

Management
Prophylaxis:
- MMR (measles, mumps, rubella) vaccine
- passive immunization with gamma globulin (for those at risk)
Specific:
- nil available
- antibiotics for secondary bacterial complications

Kawasaki disease (mucocutaneous lymph node syndrome)

Definition
A feverish sporadic illness of young children due to a diffuse vasculitis of unknown aetiology having an acute febrile toxic phase affecting the mouth, eyes and skin and a subacute phase involving the joints and, more importantly, the heart in some.

Characteristics

Symptoms
An acutely ill feverish child with conjunctival infection and a rash.

Signs
Exanthem lesions:
• red, indurated palms and soles
• a pleomorphic rash of the trunk, proximal extremities and perineum resulting in desquamation during the subacute phase which follows
Enanthem lesions: dry red mouth and lips, strawberry tongue
Cervical lymphadenitis

Complications
During subacute phase:
• arthralgia and arthritis in 50%
• cardiac in 20% (overall mortality of 1%), myocarditis and aneurysm obstruction and stenosis of the coronary arteries

Diagnosis
• clinical
• no specific test

Differential diagnosis
• other exanthems
• streptococcal infection
• staphylococcal scalded skin syndrome

Management
• aspirin—anti-inflammatory doses initially and then antithrombotic
• gamma globulin—to block endothelial damage by antibodies

Orf

Definition
A cutaneous parapox infection usually of the finger contracted by direct inoculation from an infected lamb or goat and occasionally inanimate material which lasts a month and heals without sequelae.

Characteristics

Symptoms
A spot on the finger usually in a farmer, shepherd or butcher after an incubation period of 5 days.

Signs
Lesions: a progression from a red or purple papule to a 'target'-like nodule with a haemorrhagic crusted centre, grey-white middle and an outer zone of erythema (Fig. 11.10).

Distribution
Usually solitary on a finger.

Complications
• lymphangiitis and regional adenitis
• occasionally erythema multiforme

Diagnosis
• clinical
• direct visualization of the virus by electron microscopy of material from under the crust or a skin biopsy

Differential diagnosis
Herpes simplex.

Management
• nil specific
• antibiotics if necessary for secondary bacterial infection

Human immunodeficiency virus (cutaneous manifestations)

Definition
An infection with a retrovirus with an affinity for CD4 T-lymphocytes resulting in immunosuppression (and consequently opportunistic infections) accompanied by neurological and neoplastic disorders. It is transmitted via infected semen or blood or transplacentally. There are numerous cutaneous complications.

Cutaneous manifestations

Viral infections
• herpes simplex
• herpes zoster
• oral hairy leukoplakia
• molluscum contagiosum

- cytomegalovirus
- warts

Fungal infections
- candidosis
- pityriasis versicolor
- dermatophytes

Bacterial infections
- atypical mycobacteria

Infestations
- scabies, especially Norwegian scabies

Malignancy
- Kaposi's sarcoma (Fig. 11.12)
- squamous cell carcinoma

Inflammatory skin disorders
- seborrhoeic dermatitis
- psoriasis and Reiter's syndrome
- eosinophilic folliculitis
- papulopruritic eruption

Drug eruptions
- exanthems and bullous
- photosensitivity

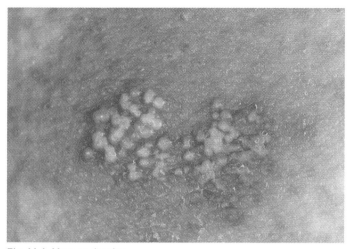

Fig. 11.1 Herpes simplex
The vesicles occur in a group on an erythematous background. The fluid is initially clear, and then becomes turbid and subsequently crusted.

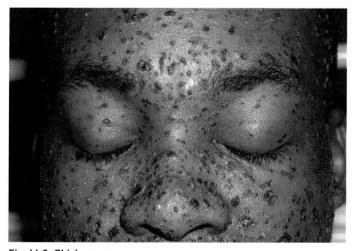

Fig. 11.2 Chickenpox
The lesions tend to occur in crops so that they are found at different stages of development. Here there are fresh vesicles particularly on the forehead, a vesiculopustule on the left cheek and numerous scabbed lesions. The distribution is centripetal, i.e. torso predominantly, then face and thighs and upper arms more than shins and forearms. Chickenpox confers lasting immunity. It remains dormant in sensory nerve ganglion cells but subsequently may reactivate as shingles and is caused by the varicella zoster (VZ) virus.

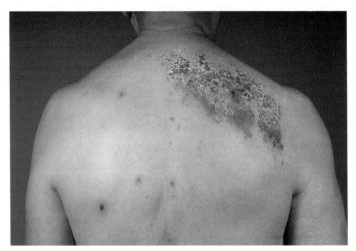

Fig. 11.3 Herpes zoster
The eruption stops at the midline, is unilateral and corresponds to the distribution of a sensory nerve. Although cellulitis is also usually unilateral, there is a diffuse erythema and oedema and not clusters of vesicles as in shingles.

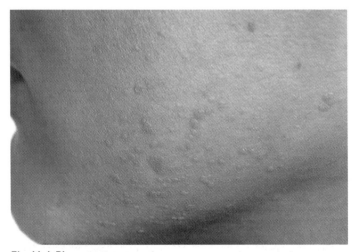

Fig. 11.4 Plane warts
There are innumerable flesh-coloured and pigmented flat-topped papules, some of which have coalesced giving an impression of a linear arrangement (Koebner phenomenon). They are often misdiagnosed and may be mistaken for acne, or worse eczema, and be treated with topical steroids. The face is a common site.

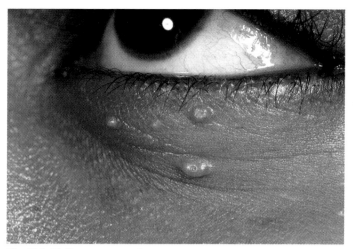

Fig. 11.5 Molluscum contagiosum
Small dome-shaped flesh-coloured papules with a central depression on the surface are present. Although the lesions ultimately will disappear spontaneously, minimal cryotherapy with liquid nitrogen is effective. This may be the presenting cutaneous sign of HIV infection.

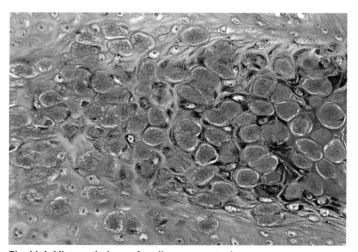

Fig. 11.6 Histopathology of molluscum contagiosum
There is a mass of homogenous round bodies in the cytoplasm of the epidermis. These inclusion bodies can be seen just as well by scraping cells off the lesion with a blunt scalpel, putting them on a microscopic slide, applying potash and viewing them under the microscope.

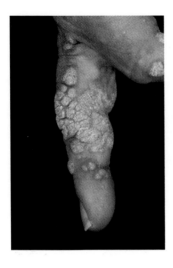

Fig. 11.7 Warts in the immunosuppressed

An enormous number of common warts are present on the fingers of this patient who was on immuno-suppressants (steroids, azathioprine and cyclosporine) following a renal transplant. Probably 80% of these · patients develop warts, mainly HPV 2 or 4.

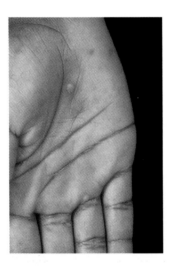

Fig. 11.8 Hand, foot and mouth disease

There are a few oval white vesicles to be found on the palms and soles, and around the digits and nails. The diagnosis is made on this distribution and involvement of the mouth. It is caused by a Coxsackie, usually A16, infection.

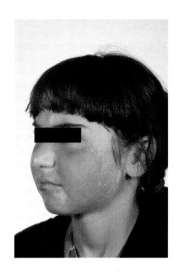

Fig. 11.9 Erythema infectiosum
There is a sudden appearance of a rash on the face and limbs without a prodrome. The facial eruption is characteristic in that it is a hot, turgid, blotchy erythema which looks almost as if the cheeks have been slapped. It is caused by the human parvovirus B19. Polyarthritis may occur in adults and cause fetal abnormalities in pregnancy.

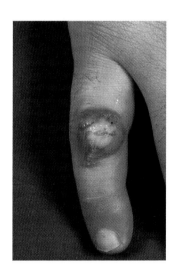

Fig. 11.10 Orf
The lesion is target-like, having a haemorrhagic crusted centre, greyish white middle and an outer zone of erythema and blistering. It is a parapoxvirus infection usually inoculated into the finger from contact with an infected lamb or goat.

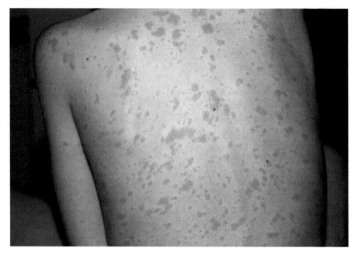

Fig. 11.11 Measles
The presence of fever, malaise, catarrh, cough and conjunctivitis is
followed by a dull red blotchy papular rash which begins on the face
and spreads to the trunk and limbs.

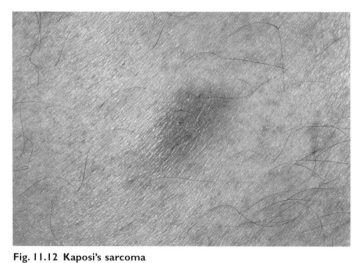

Fig. 11.12 Kaposi's sarcoma
The lesion is a purple smooth-surfaced plaque. It is a neoplasm of
endothelial cells. There is a mass of spindle cells and poorly formed vascular spaces.

12 Infestations

Scabies

Definition
A contagious eruption caused by *Sarcoptes scabiei*, a mite which lays her eggs in a burrow in the stratum corneum and induces an intensely itchy allergic response.

Characteristics

Symptoms
Itching, which is worse when warm, particularly at night, and may interfere with sleep.

Signs (see Table 12.1)

Variants
Norwegian scabies

Diagnosis
Extraction of the acarus (mite) from a burrow (Fig. 12.4).

Table 12.1 Scabies—the signs

The cause	
Lesions	Burrows—a serpiginous track with a black dot at its head (Fig. 12.1)
Distribution	Especially palmar sides of fingers, wrists, palms and soles (Fig. 12.2)
The allergic response	
1 Lesions	Small red papules often excoriated (Fig. 12.3)
Distribution	Trunk, limbs and between the fingers (Fig. 12.5)
2 Lesions	Papules or nodules
Distribution	Penis (Fig. 12.6), groin, hips, axillae, elbows
The reaction to scratching	
1 Lesions	Excoriations and bruising
Distribution	Limbs
2 Lesions	A patchy eczema
Distribution	Limbs

Differential diagnosis
- none necessary if acarus demonstrated
- eczema
- lichen planus
- insect bites
- other causes of itching

Management
- gamma benzene hexachloride
- benzyl benzoate
- malathion
- permethrin
- treatment of contacts

Pediculosis

Definition
An infestation with a louse which may be found in the pubic hair (*Phthirus pubis*) or scalp, beard and eyelashes (*Pediculus humanus*). Occasionally the latter affects all the body.

Characteristics

Symptoms
Itching.

Signs and distribution
The presence of lice and nits:
- in the scalp hair—head louse
- in the pubic hair—pubic louse (Fig. 12.7)
- in the clothing—body louse

The presence of:
- urticated papules on the back of the neck—head lice
- widespread excoriations and blood on the clothing—body lice

Diagnosis
Identification of a louse or nit.

Differential diagnosis
- unnecessary once nit or louse identified
- other causes of itching

Management
- gamma benzene hexachloride
- malathion

Insect bites

Definition
An itchy papular or urticarial response to a biting or stinging arthopod, which sometimes acts to transmit diseases such as malaria (mosquitoes), leishmaniasis (sand flies) and Rocky Mountain spotted fever (ticks).

Characteristics

Symptoms
Itchy spots.

Signs
Red, urticated papules or wheals, occasionally vesicles or bullae often with a red central punctum or excoriated surface.

Distribution
• arranged in groups
• asymmetrical or exposed skin especially lower legs and ankles

Associations
Arthropods as vectors of disease, such as:
• Lyme disease
• cutaneous leishmaniasis

Diagnosis
• clinical
• occasional biopsy
• brushings from pets for microscopy
• examination of lodgings or place of work by a pest control agency

Differential diagnosis
• other itchy skin conditions
• delusional parasitophobia

Management
• elimination of the source
• symptomatic treatment
• calamine
• crotamiton/hydrocortisone in combination
• systemic antihistamines
• systemic antibiotics (if secondarily infected)

Larva migrans

Definition
An infestation with the larvae of a hookworm usually acquired through the skin from contact with soil or sand contaminated by dog faeces.

Characteristics

Symptoms
An itchy slowly moving track, often found after a beach holiday.

Signs
One or several linear mobile serpiginous tracks (Fig. 12.8)

Distribution
Usually on the buttock, hand or ankle (skin in contact with sand).

Diagnosis
Clinical and unmistakable.

Management
- albendazole 400 mg daily for 3 days, *or*
- application of 10% thiabendazole (two 0.5 g tablets in 10 g petrolatum or equivalent base) twice daily for 10 days

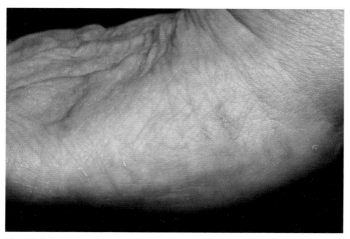

Fig. 12.1 Scabies

There are burrows in the palmar skin near the wrist. The black dot at the end of the burrow represents the gravid mite, which can be extracted with a needle. The mite attaches herself to it and can be put onto a slide and demonstrated under a microscope. The stratum corneum is thickest in palmar and plantar skin which is ideal for the mite to burrow into.

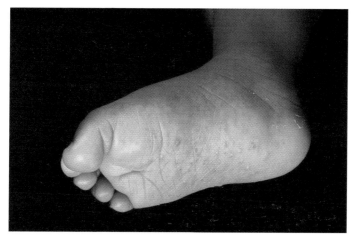

Fig. 12.2 Scabies

In infancy burrows are particularly to be found on the soles of the feet, and may be vesicular. The baby is frequently seen to rub the feet together to relieve the itching. Babies acquire scabies from people who hold them in their arms like their mothers and nannies and may clearly pass it on to other relatives and friends.

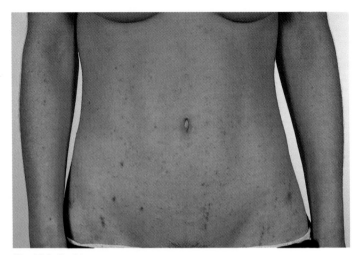

Fig. 12.3 Scabies
The presence of the mite induces an allergic response about a month later. This is manifest as a papular eruption which insidiously becomes highly pruritic especially when the subject is warm, after a bath or in bed at night and excoriations may be marked. The mite is transmitted from one person to another by prolonged physical contact, for example by sharing the same bed, but not by social contact such as shaking hands.

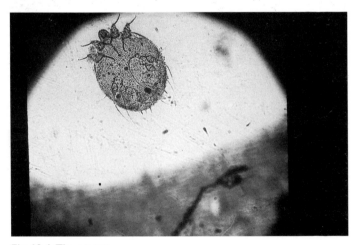

Fig. 12.4 The acarus
Scabies is caused by an acarus which is an eight-legged mite. It is seldom necessary to perform a biopsy to show the mite, since it can be extracted with a pin.

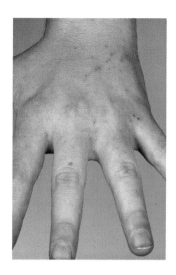

Fig. 12.5 Scabies
Papules occur between the finger webs. Burrows may be formed along the sides of the fingers and on the palms, especially the hypo- and hyperthenar eminences.

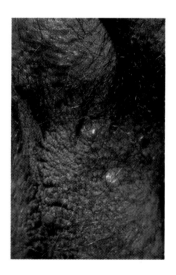

Fig. 12.6 Scabies
Papules or nodules on the penis or scrotum are usually present in scabies and aid the diagnosis. These often persist for several weeks, occasionally longer, after successful treatment with gamma benzene hexachloride or malathion. Treatment of scabies is not easy. The applications must be performed thoroughly and on two occasions only. Although the itching improves, it does not disappear completely for up to 4 weeks.

155

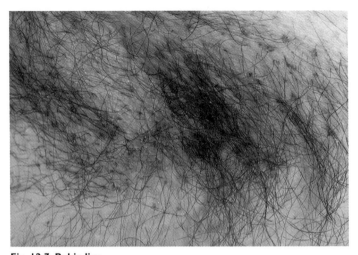

Fig. 12.7 Pubic lice
The complaint is of considerable irritation in the pubic area. Careful examination is necessary to identify the nits attached to the pubic hairs and the crab lice.

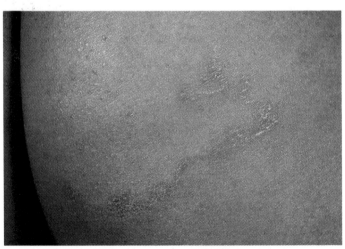

Fig. 12.8 Larva migrans
There is a linear circuitous track which the patient describes as slowly mobile. It is due to hookworm larvae, from the faeces of an infected dog, which penetrate human skin that is in contact with contaminated soil—usually sand on a Caribbean or Floridan beach.

13 Acne and Rosacea

Acne

Definition
A chronic disorder of the pilosebaceous apparatus associated with excess production of grease (sebum), bacterial overgrowth particularly of *Propionobacteria acnes* and blockage of the pilosebaceous duct resulting in a variety of inflammatory manifestations on the face and torso.

Characteristics

Symptoms
Spot under the skin which may be itchy or painful.

Signs
Lesions:
- comedones (blackheads)
- milia (whiteheads)
- red papules
- pustules
- red nodules
- cysts
- scars
- keloids
- hyperpigmented macules
- some or all of the above

Distribution
One site often predominates:
- face
- back
- front of chest

Types
- acne vulgaris
- infantile acne
- mature female's acne (Fig. 13.1)
- acne conglobata (nodulocystic acne) (Fig. 13.3)
- steroid-induced acne (Fig. 13.2)
- occlusive (pommade, tropical humidity, oils and clothing)
- caused by drugs/chemicals (progestogens, anti-oestrogens, halogens)
- caused by alcohol

Table 13.1 Drug-induced causes of acne

Hormones	
Steroids	Endogenous (Cushing's)
	Exogenous
	Systemic
	Topical
Anti-oestrogens	e.g. tamoxifen
Progestogens	Oral contraceptives
	HRT
	Premenstrual
	e.g. danazol
Androgens	
Halogens	
Chloracne	
Iodides	Cough mixture
	Seaweed
	Radiological contrast materials
Bromides	Treatment of thyroid disease
Other drugs	Phenobarbitone
	Troxidone
	Isoniazid

Associations
Hidradenitis suppurativa (Fig. 13.5).

Differential diagnosis
Not usually a problem except for itchy mild acne being misdiagnosed as eczema.
- rosacea
- acne excoriée des jeunes filles

Treatment

Topical
Antibacterials/keratolytics/retinoic acid.

Systemic
- long-term antibiotics
- anti-androgens (Dianette) for females only
- isotretinoin (Roaccutane) (13-*cis*-retinoic acid) (Fig. 13.4)

Rosacea

Definition
A disorder of flushing of the skin of the face resulting in erythema, papules and pustules especially on the forehead, cheeks, nose and chin sometimes associated with rhinophyma, periorbital lymphoedema and ocular disorders.

Characteristics

Symptoms
Spots on the face and flushing.

Signs (Fig. 13.6)
• papules
• pustules
• erythema and telangiectasia

Distribution
• forehead
• cheeks
• nose
• chin

Special features
• rhinophyma (Fig. 13.7)
• periorbital lymphoedema
• ocular complications (e.g. conjunctivitis, blepharitis and keratitis)

Variants
• red nose (Fig. 13.8)
• steroid-modified rosacea

Associations
Alcohol abuse.

Differential diagnosis
Acne vulgaris (Table 13.2).

Treatment
• low-dose long-term oral antibiotics, especially tetracylines (including minocycline and doxycycline) and erythromycin
• topical sulphur or metronidazole
• 13-*cis*-retinoic acid (Isotretinoin, Roaccutane) in recalcitrant cases.

Table 13.2 Distinguishing features of acne from rosacea

Acne
Onset in youth
Greasiness
Comedones, milia, cysts, scars, nodules and pustules
Slow response to antibiotics

Rosacea
Later onset
Erythema and flushing
Papules and pustules only
Rapid response to antibiotics

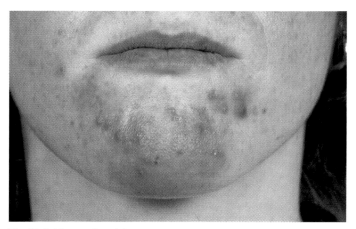

Fig. 13.1 Mature female's acne
This variety occurs in women in their 20s or 30s who had no acne during adolescence. It affects the jaw and chin (female equivalent of the beard area). It is often worse premenstrually. It may be associated with low sex hormone binding levels resulting in raised levels of free circulating testosterone and with the polycystic ovary syndrome. The anti-androgen, cyproterone acetate, coupled with ethinyl oestradiol (Dianette) may be particularly helpful.

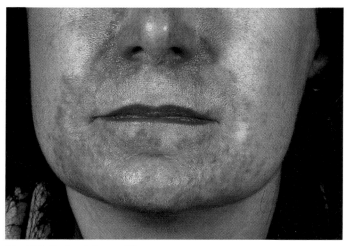

Fig. 13.2 Perioral dermatitis
This term is a misnomer because dermatitis is absent and perioral papules are present. This condition usually results from the erroneous treatment of mild (often mature female premenstrual) acne with topical steroids. It responds to conventional treatment with oral antibiotics or Dianette.

161

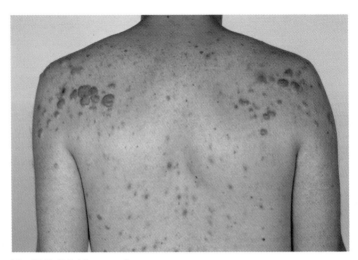

Fig. 13.3 Keloids secondary to acne
In severe forms of acne vulgaris and in all forms of acne conglobata
scarring occurs. In some cases this scarring may take the form of keloids
such as these overlying the scapulae. They may be treated with variable
degrees of success with triamcinolone injected via an insulin syringe.

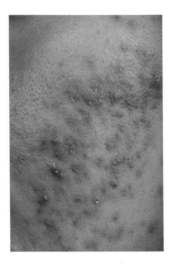

**Fig. 13.4 Roaccutane treatment
of acne**
This 25-year-old woman had
intractable scarring acne, unrespon-
sive to systemic antibiotics or anti-
androgens. She was commenced on
13-*cis*-retinoic acid in a dose of 1
mg/kg body weight for 16 weeks,
whilst continuing on her oral con-
traceptive because it is a teratogen.
Normal liver function is a prerequi-
site for its prescription.

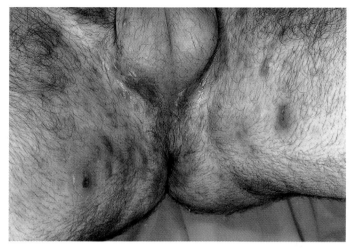

Fig. 13.5 Hidradenitis suppurativa
This is a chronic inflammatory disorder either of the apocrine glands, which develop as part of the pilosebaceous follicle in the embryo or of the hair follicle. They localize to the axillae, areolae and perianal region, enlarging with androgen stimulation at puberty. They secrete an oily fluid. Indolent painful pustules and nodules which result in scarring and sinus formation occur in the axillae, groin and buttocks and around the anus. It often occurs in association with acne conglobata. Pathogens are rarely recovered. Long-term antibiotics and Roaccutane may be tried but with varied success. Excision and grafting is effective in severe cases particularly in the axillae.

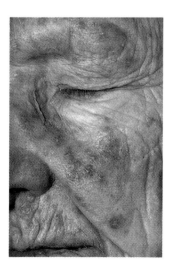

Fig. 13.6 Rosacea
The physical signs are pustules associated with erythema, telangiectasia and flushing. Comedones, cysts and scarring which occur in acne do not in rosacea. Topical steroids must not be used. Small doses of antibiotics taken over several months are effective but relapse is not uncommon.

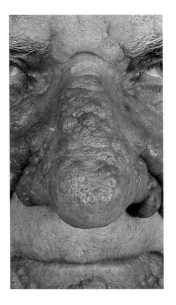

Fig. 13.7 Rhinophyma
There is sebaceous gland hypertrophy and overgrowth of the soft tissues resulting in a bulbous nose. It may occur in association with rosacea or in isolation. The glands may be surgically pared away and the nose remodelled to produce an effective cosmetic result.

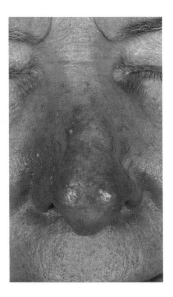

Fig. 13.8 Rosacea
The erythema may be striking and surmounted by papules and pustules. It is exacerbated by alcohol, hot drinks and sunlight.

14 Hair and Scalp Disorders

Pityriasis amiantacea

Definition
A common disorder of the scalp characterized by thick white scales which adhere to the hair and may result in a minor temporary loss of hair. It is usually secondary to seborrhoeic eczema or psoriasis.

Characteristics

Symptoms
A scalp condition which appears resistant to commonly used shampoos or topical steroids.

Signs
Thick scales adhering to the base of the hair shaft (Fig. 14.1).

Distribution
The scalp.

Diagnosis
A distinctive morphological appearance.

Differential diagnosis
• seborrhoeic eczema
• psoriasis
• tinea capitis (Fig. 14.2)

Treatment
Tar and salicylic acid ointment (cocois).

Trichotillomania

Definition
Hair loss due to mechanical interference by the patient which is a common neurotic temporary disturbance of childhood but occasionally occurs in adult life in association with depression or psychosis and is persistent.

Characteristics

Symptoms
Localized hair loss.

Signs

One (usually) or more asymmetrical patches of hair loss without inflammation. The hairs are broken off at varying lengths above the surface.

Distribution

One side of the scalp usually corresponding with the handedness of the patient (Fig. 14.3).

Differential diagnosis

Localized hair loss occurring in children (Table 14.1).

Treatment

• reassurance in children
• treatment of underlying psychosis or depression in adults

Table 14.1 Possible causes of hair loss in children

	Hair loss	Inflammation	Scarring
Tinea capitis (Fig. 10.1)	One or several patches	Yes	Not usual
Pityriasis amantacea (Fig. 14.2)	Not obviously until treatment	Yes with especially thick scales	No
Alopecia areata (Fig. 18.2)	Total loss in round patches	No	No
Discoid lupus erythematosus	One or several patches	Yes	Yes
Traction	Corresponding with tension on hair roots	No	Occasionally
Trichotillomania (Fig. 14.3)	Patchy partial and asymmetrical	No	No

Table 14.2 Causes of generalized hair loss

Androgenetic alopecia
Telogen effluvium (Fig. 14.4; Table 14.3)
Endocrine
  hypo- and hyperthyroidism
  hypopituitarism
  hypoparathyroidism
Infection
  including syphilis
Alopecia universalis
Lupus erythematosus
Malnutrition
  including malabsorption and iron and zinc deficiency
Drugs
  cytotoxics (especially cyclophosphamide)
  anticoagulants
  thyroid antagonists
  retinoids including excess vitamin A
  X-rays

Table 14.3 Causes of telogen effluvium (Fig. 14.4)

Feverish illness (including influenza)
Surgery
Haemorrhage (including blood donation)
Post partum
Crash dieting
Following any illness (including depression)

Table 14.4 Causes of hirsutism

Constitutional/racial
Increased production of ovarian androgens
  polycystic ovaries
  ovarian tumours
Ovarian failure
  postoophorectomy
  postmenopausal
Increased production of adrenal androgens
  adrenal tumours or hyperplasia
  hyperpituitarism
Inborn error of steroid metabolism
  adrenogenital syndrome
Androgenic drugs
  testosterone
  danazol
  progestogens
  systemic steroids

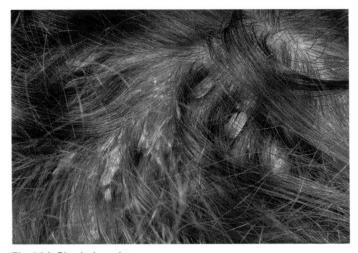

Fig. 14.1 Pityriasis amiantacea
Thick scales are seen attached to the lower part of the shaft of the hair.
It may be caused by psoriasis or seborrheic dermatitis. It responds to tar-
containing ointments.

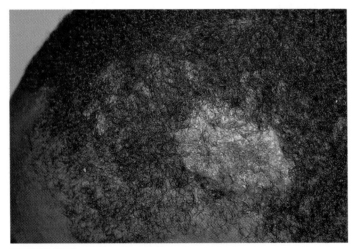

Fig. 14.2 Kerion
If the inflammatory response is marked (as in Trichophyton tonsurans
here), the clinical appearance is known as a kerion. Tinea capitis only
responds to oral antifungal agents.

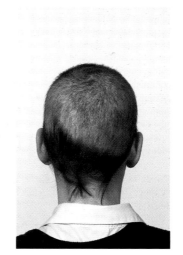

Fig. 14.3 Trichotillomania

This is not uncommon in childhood, when it is a habit tic (rather like nail biting) and is a temporary abnormality of minor psychological significance. The hair loss is partial and asymmetrical with the hairs broken off at different lengths. It occasionally occurs in adults and tends to be more persistent.

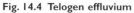

Fig. 14.4 Telogen effluvium

This young woman's hair fell out precipitously 3 months after a severe pustular skin eruption secondary to amoxycillin. The hair has completely regrown 3 months later. The loss is diffuse and includes the sides and back of the scalp. Any severe illness may do this. It is due to a premature precipitation of anagen (actively growing) hairs into catagen (a resting phase) which lasts 3 months, after which the hairs all fall out.

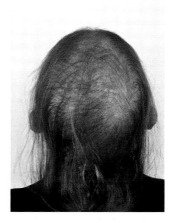

15   Pigmentary Disorders

Causes of generalized hyperpigmentation
- ultraviolet irradiation
- hormonal (increased production of ACTH and MSH)
- chronic infection (e.g. tuberculosis)
- scleroderma
- liver disease (especially primary biliary cirrhosis and haemochromatosis)
- chronic renal insufficiency
- malabsorption and nutritional deficiencies (including vitamin B_{12})
- neoplasia (especially carcinoma of the bronchus and lymphoma)
- common drugs
  - —psoralens
  - —busulphan
  - —cyclophosphamide
  - —arsenic
  - —chlorpromazine

Melasma (chloasma)

Definition
A patchy brown hyperpigmentation of face, especially the forehead, cheeks, upper lip, chin and jaw, due to solar damage but enhanced by pregnancy and oestrogens, more common in women who tan easily but also occurring in dark skinned races in both sexes.

Characteristics

Symptoms
An unsightly discoloration on the face, which is darkened by sunlight.

Signs
An ill-defined patchy, flat, brown pigmentation (Fig. 15.1).

Distribution
The face, fairly symmetrically distributed on the forehead, cheeks, bridge of nose, upper lip (simulating a moustache), chin and jaw.

Associations
- pregnancy
- oral contraceptives

Differential diagnosis
- Poikiloderma of Civatte
- fixed drug eruption
- phototoxicity
- ochronosis (Fig. 15.2)

Treatment
- complete avoidance of ultraviolet irradiation
- sunblocks
- hats
- stop oestrogens
- 2% hydroquinone and 0.05% retinoic acid in 1% hydrocortisone cream as a depigmenting agent (not very satisfactory)

Causes of generalized hypopigmentation
Hormonal:
- hypopituitarism (melanocyte-stimulating hormone deficiency)

Failure of melanin production:
- albinism
- phenylketonuria

Absence of melanocytes:
- generalized vitiligo
- piebaldism

Pityriasis alba

Definition
A patchy, partial loss of pigment affecting the face in childhood and adolescence which is thought to be post-inflammatory (possibly due to eczema) and is persistent although it ultimately disappears.

Characteristics

Symptoms
Loss of pigment on the face.

Signs
Ill-defined patches of hypopigmentation.

Distribution
Face, especially cheeks (Fig. 15.3).

Differential diagnosis

- vitiligo (Fig. 15.4)
- pityriasis versicolor

Management

- nil specific
- photoprotection in Caucasians

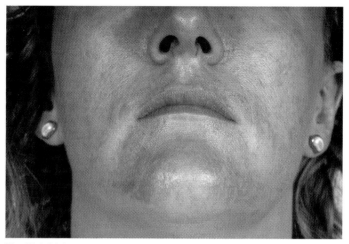

Fig. 15.1 Melasma

This is a patchy pigmentation on the face. It occurs in both sexes and is exacerbated by ultraviolet irradiation. There is a hormonal and racial (common in people from Asian and Mediterranean countries) component. Treatment is unsatisfactory. Obsessional avoidance of sunlight is mandatory.

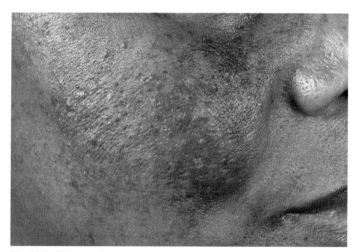

Fig. 15.2 Ochronosis

This occurs on the face, particularly over bony prominences, as an adverse reaction in people with black skin (usually Africans) who use hydroquinones to bleach or lighten the skin.

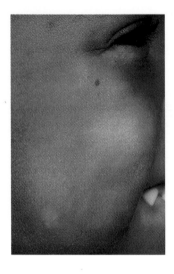

Fig. 15.3 Pityriasis alba
There is a patchy, partial loss of pigmentation mainly on the cheeks. It occurs in childhood, is very common in pigmented skins and is persistent, but ultimately clears spontaneously.

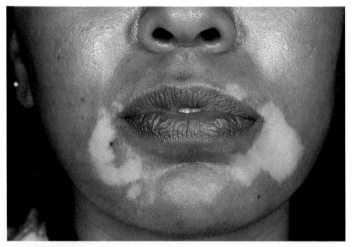

Fig. 15.4 Vitiligo
There is complete loss of pigment (depigmentation) and the skin is white in colour. It is usually symmetrical.

16 Nail Disorders

Physical signs

Pitting

Definition
Small depressions in the nail plate which may be scattered or arranged in lines.

Causes
- alopecia areata (Fig. 16.5)
- psoriasis
- eczema
- 20-nail dystrophy of childhood

Ridging of the nails

Definition
A visible horizontal or vertical line across or along the nail plate resulting from a disturbance in nail growth.

Causes
Horizontal:
- inflammatory disorders affecting the nail folds, e.g. eczema, candida
- Beau's lines

Vertical:
- median nail dystrophy (Fig. 16.1)
- habit tic

Lamellar dystrophy

Definition
A splitting of the distal end of the nail plate into its constituent layers (Fig. 16.2).

Causes
Water damage to the nail plate.

Abnormally curved nails

Definition
A curving of the nail plate either horizontally, vertically or concavely.

Common causes
- koilonychia
- clubbing
- ingrowing toenails
- onychogryphosis

Disturbances of colour

Causes
White:
- trauma
- tinea (Fig. 16.3)
- liver and renal disease (Fig. 16.4)
Yellow:
- psoriasis
- tinea
- yellow nail syndrome
Green:
- *Pseudomonas*
Brown:
- *Candida*
- linear melanonychia (Fig. 16.6)
Black:
- malignant melanoma (Fig. 16.7)
- tinea
- trauma
Red/brown:
- trauma

Onycholysis

Definition
Separation of the nail away from the nail bed.

Causes
- idiopathic (Fig. 16.8)
- tinea (Fig. 16.9)
- psoriasis (Fig. 16.13)
- phototoxicity
- thyroid disorders

Common disorders in and around the nail

Infections
- staphylococcal
- herpes simplex
- tinea

- *Candida albicans* (Fig. 16.10)
- warts

Inflammatory
- psoriasis (Fig. 16.11)
- sarcoidosis (Fig. 16.12)
- lichen planus (Fig. 16.14)
- collagen vascular disorders (Fig. 16.15)
- eczema

Tumours

Benign
- subungual exostosis (Fig. 16.16)
- myxoid cyst (Fig. 16.17)
- pyogenic granuloma

Malignant
- squamous cell carcinoma
- malignant melanoma
- clubbing (Fig. 16.18 and Table 16.1)

Table 16.1 Causes of clubbing

Pulmonary
Carcinoma of the bronchus
Mesothelioma
Bronchiectasis
Tuberculosis
Fibrosing alveolitis

Cardiac
Subacute bacterial endocarditis
Congenital cyanotic heart disease

Others
Crohn's disease
Ulcerative colitis
Thyrotoxicosis
Cirrhosis

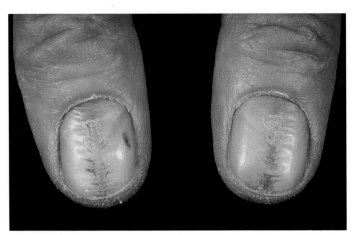

Fig. 16.1 Median canal dystrophy
This condition affects the thumb nails only. The lunulae are prominent.
There are small lines extending outward from the central ridge or split
giving the impression of an inverted fir tree. It is possibly caused by
trauma. The condition may recover after but relapse is not uncommon.

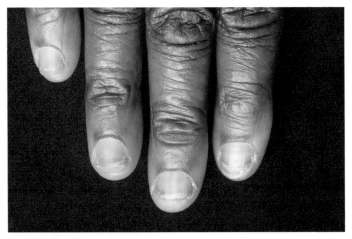

Fig. 16.2 Lamellar nail dystrophy
This is common in females who get their hands wet a lot. The distial nail
is softened by water and consequently splits into its constituent layers.

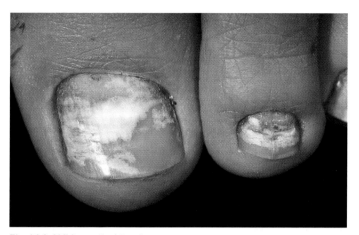

Fig. 16.3 White nails (tinea)
A patchy white discoloration is present in the nails without much evidence of the thickening or soft subungual hyperkeratosis which is usually present in onychomycosis (dermatophyte infection). This distinctive form of white superficial tinea is commonly caused by *Trichophyton interdigitale*.

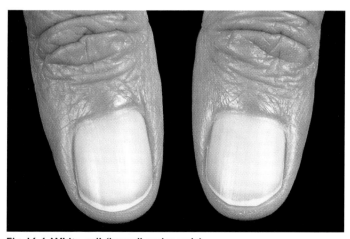

Fig. 16.4 White nail (hypoalbuminaemia)
The nail bed may be pale causing a total leuconychia in association with hypoalbuminaemia due either to renal, or as in this case, to liver disease.

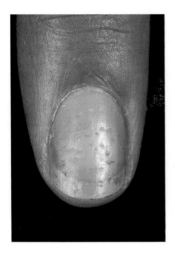

Fig. 16.5 Pitting
Scattered pits are present in the nail plate. It is sometimes associated with alopecia areata (particularly universalis) but psoriasis is the most common cause.

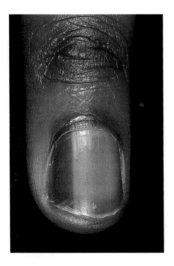

Fig. 16.6 Linear melanonychia
A well-defined straight, broad black band may involve one or more nails. Sometimes the whole nail is discoloured. This is common in Blacks but less so in Caucasians. Trauma or a melanocytic naevus at the nail matrix may be the cause.

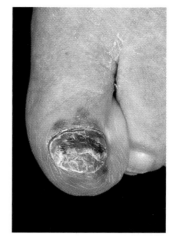

Fig. 16.7 Malignant melanoma
There is a loss of the distal portion
of the nail due to a red nodule
underneath. The rest of the
melanoma is at an earlier stage and
has produced some elevation of the
proximal nail with pigmentation of
varying shades of dark brown and
black, and involvement of the surrounding skin (Hutchinson's sign).

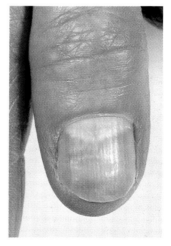

Fig. 16.8 Onycholysis (traumatic)
There is separation of the nail away
from the nail bed, and superinfec-
tion with *Pseudomonas*. This is a condition of women who tend to keep
their nails long. Minor trauma tears
the projecting part of the nail away
from the nail bed. Reattachment
usually takes place if the nail is kept
cut short.

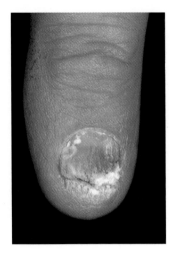

Fig. 16.9 Onycholysis (tinea)
There is loss of the distal part of the nail following onycholysis, which is still visible. The nail plate is thickened and discolored. Tinea affecting the finger nails is remarkable for usually involving one hand only. However, both sets of toe nails are normally infected first.

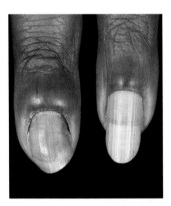

Fig. 16.10 Candida of the nail
The cuticle is softened and destroyed by constant immersion in water (e.g. cooks, domestics, nurses, etc.). Candida then gains entry under the posterior nail fold which becomes swollen. The nail growth is disturbed with horizontal ridging and nail plate discoloured if invaded by candida. The nail must be kept dry (not covered) and treated with a topical and sometimes systemic imidazole.

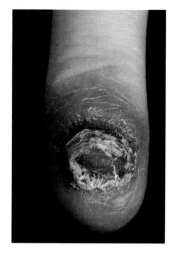

Fig. 16.11 Psoriasis
Psoriasis underneath and surrounding the nail interferes with nail growth such that it may thicken, and subsequently detach from the underlying nail bed. Treatment is unsatisfactory. Intralesional steroids are sometimes tried. Systemic agents are effective but not usually indicated.

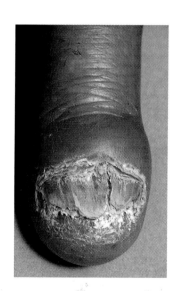

Fig. 16.12 Sarcoidosis
The whole of the distal phalanx is swollen and the nail is discoloured, slightly thickening and split. Bony cysts and erosions are found on X-ray.

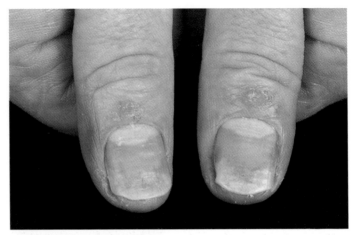

Fig. 16.13 Onycholysis (psoriasis)
The distal part of both thumb nails have separated from the nail bed. Psoriasis is present at the posterior nail fold which reinforces the diagnosis, but the yellow margin between the normal pink nail and the onycholysis is rather characteristic of psoriasis as is the symmetry.

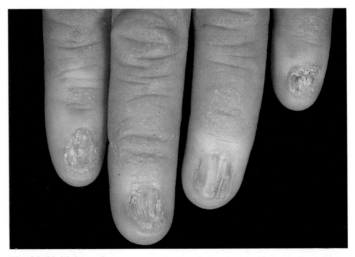

Fig. 16.14 Lichen planus
Lichen planus rarely affects the nails but when it does it causes scarring such that the nail is destroyed and the skin of the posterior nail fold grows forward onto the nail forming a pterygium (a wing-like process).

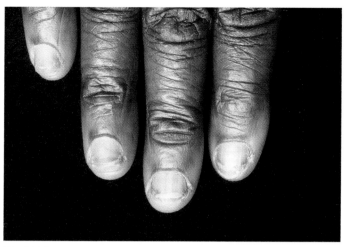

Fig. 16.15 Dermatomyiasis
Characteristically there is a purple discolouration over the inter-
phalangeal joints and around the nails. The cuticles are ragged and
haemorrhages are common.

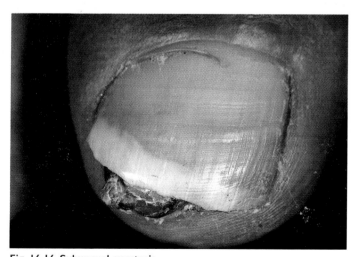

Fig. 16.16 Subungual exostosis
The distal edge of the nail is lifted up by a discrete firm swelling. X-ray
reveals an area of calcification. Excision is curative.

185

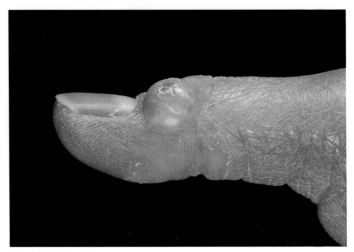

Fig. 16.17 Myxoid cyst
There is a flesh-coloured swelling over the distal phalanx or inter-
phalangeal joint. It results from degeneration of the connective tissue. It
causes a characteristic furrow along the nail and a gelatinous discharge.
It can be excised but may recur.

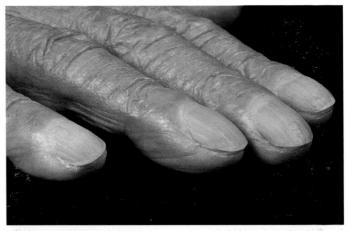

Fig. 16.18 Clubbing
The angle between the nail and the posterior nail fold should be less
than 180°. (The nail is described as clubbed when the angle is equal to
or greater than 180°.) Subsequently the distal phalanx becomes enlarged
and with it the nail. The common causes are shown in Table 16.1.

17 Developmental Disorders

Ichthyosis vulgaris

Definition
A chronic widespread non-inflammatory scaling of the skin, inherited as an autosomal dominant trait, usually present at birth and often associated with atopic eczema.

Characteristics

Symptoms
Dry skin, which is worse in the winter and improves in the summer.

Signs
Small fine white scales (although larger and more prominent on the shins) (Fig. 17.1).

Distribution
Extensor surfaces sparing the flexures especially knees and elbows.

Associations
• atopic eczema
• keratosis pilaris

Differential diagnosis
• X-linked ichthyosis vulgaris (see below)
• acquired ichthyosis

Management
• oils and emollients
• topical steroids for associated eczema only

X-linked ichthyosis vulgaris

Definition
An uncommon X-linked recessive inherited disorder resulting in a generalized abnormality of large dark scales on the skin due to a steroid sulphatase deficiency. It occurs only in males whose mothers often have a prolonged labour due to placental steroid sulphatase deficiency.

Characteristics

Symptoms
A dry, rather dirty-looking skin.

Signs
Large, dark, rough scales (Fig. 17.2).

Distribution
Universal.

Associations
- corneal opacities
- cryptorchidism

Diagnosis
- clinical
- measure steroid sulphatase

Differential diagnosis
Ichthyosis vulgaris (see above).

Management
- nil specific
- emollients
- occasionally oral retinoids

Keratosis pilaris

Definition
A common disorder of keratinization of the skin around the exit of the hair shaft on the extensor surfaces of the upper arms and thighs resulting in discrete small rough papules in adolescence and often persisting into adult life if inherited as an autosomal dominant.

Characteristics

Symptoms
Goose flesh.

Signs
Small, rough, horny papules sometimes surrounded by erythema.

Distribution
- posterolateral aspects of upper arms and thighs (Fig. 17.3)
- occasionally buttocks
- occasionally on the cheeks

Associations
- physiological in 50% of adolescents
- rarely in gross nutritional and vitamin A deficiency (phrynoderma)
- atopy

Differential diagnosis
Not usually necessary.

Management
Nil specific.

Palmar plantar keratoderma

Definition
A markedly thickened palmar and plantar skin, either associated with other ectodermal defects or acquired, usually affecting most of the surface but occasionally punctuate especially in black-skinned people.

Characteristics

Symptoms
Thick rough skin which may crack in cold weather and be painful.

Signs
Symmetrical, well-defined diffusely thickened skin; may be localized and punctate in black races.

Distribution
Palms and soles.

Differential diagnosis
- other acquired causes of palmar plantar keratoderma (see Table 17.1)
- other eruptions of the palms or soles

Management
- of the cause if known
- emollients

Table 17.1 Causes of palmar plantar keratoderma

Genetic
    Dominant and recessive forms
    Familial association with carcinoma of the oesophagus (tylosis)
    Associated with other genodermatoses (including Darier's disease)
Acquired
    Climacteric
    Pityriasis rubra pilaris
    Sézary syndrome
    Myxoedema
    Acanthosis nigricans
    Keratoderma blenorrhagica
    Paraneoplastic

Darier's disease

Definition
A chronic disorder of keratinization, inherited as an autosomal dominant, resulting in red–brown, slightly crusted papules particularly on the torso and face due to a failure of epidermal cells to adhere together correctly secondary to a loss of desmosomes and malfunctioning of monofilaments.

Characteristics

Symptoms
A rash on the face and trunk.

Signs
Lesions: large numbers of papules which may coalesce into plaques.
Colour: greasy yellow or red–brown (Fig. 17.4).
Surface: slightly fissured or crusted.

Distribution
The seborrhoeic areas, especially the chest and back but also the face and groin.

Associations
- nail involvement
- palmar/plantar pits
- small 'cobblestone'-like papules in the mouth
- flat wart-like papules on the backs of the hands and feet

Complications
- secondary bacterial infection
- Kaposi's varicelliform eruption

Diagnosis
- clinical
- histopathology

Differential diagnosis
Seborrhoeic eczema.

Management
- unsatisfactory
- avoidance of sunlight
- anti-infectives
- oral retinoids

Hailey–Hailey disease (benign familial chronic pemphigus)

Definition
An autosomal dominantly inherited disorder of epidermal cell adhesion with incomplete penetrance affecting the major flexures causing vesiculation and fissuring of the skin as a result of friction or sepsis, usually commencing in adolescence.

Characteristics

Symptoms
An eruption in the armpits and groin.

Signs
Vesicles which rupture readily and result in a plaque of red, partially fissured, partially crusted skin.

Distribution
Major flexures (Fig. 17.5), especially axillae and groin.

Diagnosis
- clinical
- histopathology

Differential diagnosis
Other flexural disorders (axilla/groin).

Management
- swabs for microbiology and appropriate antimicrobial agents
- topical steroid; appropriate antibiotic; anti-*Candida* preparations
- superficial X-ray therapy
- excision of affected skin and grafting

Neurofibromatosis I (von Recklinghausen's disease)

Definition
A common neurectodermal abnormality transmitted as an autosomal dominant by a gene on chromosome 17 but frequently occurring as a new mutation resulting in multiple neurofibromata, café-au-lait patches, axillary freckling and pigmented hamartomata of the iris (Lisch nodules) and potentially a legion of other organ abnormalities.

Characteristics

Symptoms
Lumps on the skin.

Signs
- café-au-lait patches
- freckles in the axillae and often other intertriginous sites
- neurofibromata (Fig. 17.6)

Distribution
Widespread.

Associations
- oral tumours and macroglossia
- kyphoscoliosis
- short stature
- macrocephaly
- endocrine abnormalities
- possible intellectual impairment
- neurofibrosarcoma

Differential diagnosis
Not usually relevant.

Management
- nil specific
- symptomatic surgery
- genetic counselling (prenatal diagnosis is possible)

Tuberous sclerosis

Definition
A variably expressed autosomal dominant disorder due to a gene or chromosome, causing hamartomata of the brain, eye, kidney and heart asso-

ciated with specific cutaneous abnormalities and sometimes with epilepsy and mental retardation.

Characteristics

Symptoms
Usually a rash on the face.

Signs and distribution (see Table 17.2)

Associations
- mental deficiency
- epilepsy
- cardiac rhabdomyomata
- renal angiomyolipomata
- endocrine abnormalities
- ocular irregularities

Diagnosis
- clinical
- Wood's light examination for ash-leaf macules
- family history
- ocular and other systemic findings including epilepsy

Differential diagnosis
Other facial eruptions (especially papular).

Management
- of the disease
- lasers for angiofibromata

Epidermolysis bullosa

Definition
A rare genetically determined collection of disorders characterized by marked fragility of the skin due to various structural defects involving the region of the basement membrane at the junction of epidermis and dermis. It results in blistering of the skin either localized to the palms and soles or generalized, and then also sometimes affecting the mucous membranes and causing scarring.

Characteristics

Symptoms
Blistering of the skin induced by minor trauma from birth (junctional and dystrophic variants) or childhood (simplex variant).

Table 17.2 Signs and distribution of tuberous sclerosis

	Signs	Distribution
Angiofibromata	Firm discrete red–brown smooth-surfaced papules which may coalesce (Fig. 17.7)	Nasolabial furrows, cheeks, nose, chin (usually appear from early childhood onwards)
Shagreen patch (connective tissue naevus)	Soft flesh-coloured plaque (Fig. 17.8)	Often over lumbar sacral region
Ovoid (ash-leaf) macule	A small ovoid off-white patch (Fig. 17.9)	On trunk or limbs (the earliest physical sign often present at birth)
Periungual fibroma	A smooth, flesh-coloured outgrowth	From the nail fold

Signs

- blisters
- erosions (Fig. 17.10)
- scarring
- milia

Distribution

Anywhere especially skin liable to trauma; may involve nails and mucous membranes.

Diagnosis

Electron microscopy.

Differential diagnosis

Other blistering disorders.

Management

No specific treatment; most cases require specialist attention.

Ehlers–Danlos syndrome

Definition

An inherited spectrum of disorders characterized particularly by defective type I or III collagen production. It results in fragile skin, which tears and bruises easily, heals poorly and is hyperelastic; fragile blood vessels (due to defective adventitia and surrounding connective tissue); and hypermobility of the joints.

Characteristics

Symptoms

Easily damaged and hyperelastic skin.

Signs

- fragile skin which bruises easily, heals poorly and results in papyraceous scars (Fig. 17.11)
- hyperextensible skin

Distribution

Universal, particularly over pressure points.

Associations (depending on type)

- hypermobile joints
- fragile blood vessels

Diagnosis

- clinical
- biochemistry

Management
- unsatisfactory
- referral to a specialist centre

Pseudoxanthoma elasticum

Definition
An inherited spectrum of disorders especially of elastic tissue but also collagen and the ground substance in the dermis and connective tissue of the media and intima of blood vessels, heart and Bruch's membrane of the eye, giving rise to characteristic cutaneous, retinal and cardiovascular changes.

Characteristics

Symptoms
May not be noticed until the skin is examined after an ocular or vascular complication.

Signs
- small yellow (pseudoxanthomatous) papules arranged in a reticular or linear manner giving a 'peau d'orange', or pebbly, cobblestone appearance
- soft, lax, slightly wrinkled, pendulous skin (Fig. 17.12)

Distribution
- sides of neck
- axillae
- elbow flexures
- groin
- abdomen

Associations
- angioid streaks
- various cardiovascular abnormalities

Diagnosis
- clinical
- skin biopsy (including normal skin if necessary)

Differential diagnosis
Not usually required.

Management
Of cardiac and ocular complications.

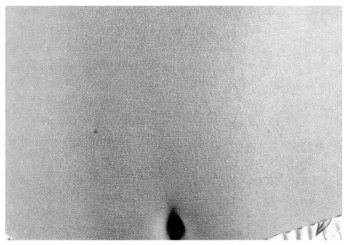

Fig. 17.1 Ichthyosis vulgaris
There are small fine white scales present without inflammation. The skin is worse in the cold and better in the warmth and humidity of summer.

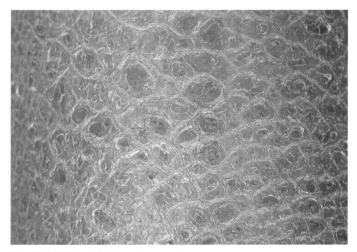

Fig. 17.2 X-linked ichthyosis vulgaris
The stratum corneum (the outermost layer of the skin) is formed at the normal rate but the cells fail to separate from each other and desquamate properly so that they shed together as collections known as plates or lamellae. There are large dark scales in X-linked ichthyosis vulgaris.

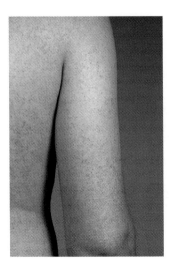

Fig. 17.3 Keratosis pilaris
This is common in adolescence and in most cases (but not in familial) it disappears. There are follicular keratotic papules on the upper arms and thighs.

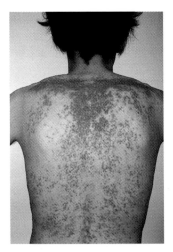

Fig. 17.4 Darier's disease
The condition is inherited as an autosomal dominant, commences in childhood and has a distribution rather similar to that of seborrhoeic dermatitis. It is due to a malformation of the tonofilament–desmosome complex, which is responsible for epidermal cell adherence. The result is that the cells separate from each other (acantholysis) resulting in fissuring within the epidermis and incorrect and premature formation of keratin.

Fig. 17.5 Hailey–Hailey disease
The disorder affects the major flexures and consists of a red plaque
composed of fissured papules and
sometimes vesicles. It is an autosomal dominant defect of epidermal
maturation probably due to a
tonofilament–desmosome complex
fault, which may be related to
Darier's disease in that the two conditions are occasionally associated. It
is exacerbated by heat, friction and
sepsis and in this case due to
contact sensitization to a medicament (neomycin).

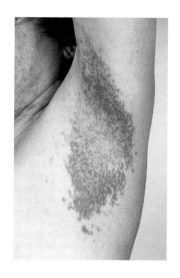

Fig. 17.6 Neurofibromatosis 1
There are numerous nodules and
papules of various sizes scattered
over the body. On examination the
neurofibromata are soft and indent
easily. Café-au-lait patches are also
visible. It is a common autosomal
dominant defect and although prenatal diagnosis is possible, genetic
counselling is difficult because the
expression varies considerably. Axillary freckles are diagnostic.

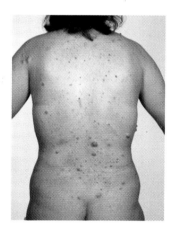

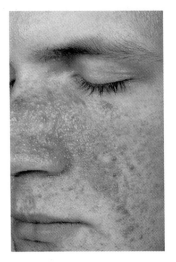

Fig. 17.7 Tuberous sclerosis
There are numerous red–brown papules spread over the nose and onto the cheeks. They appear in childhood and are known as adenoma sebaceum although histologically they are angiofibromata. The condition is sometimes known by the acronym of epiloia; epilepsy (ep), lower intelligence (loi), and adenoma sebaceum (a).

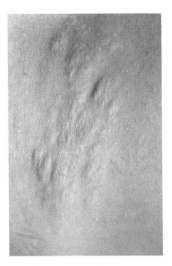

Fig. 17.8 Tuberous sclerosis
A single soft flesh-coloured plaque more raised in some areas than others and with an orange peel-like puckered surface (peau d'orange) is usually found somewhere on the skin but often over the lumbar sacral region. It is inherited as an autosomal dominant disorder but the degree of abnormality varies considerably, there being formes frustes with minor facial changes and no other conspicuous abnormality. CT scan is helpful diagnostically (even in infancy) because intraventricular calcified nodules are characteristic.

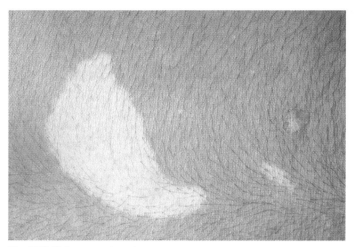

Fig. 17.9 Tuberous sclerosis
An ovoid ash-leaf patch is the first cutaneous sign to appear in life and
may help to explain the aetiology of epileptic fits in an infant. The
hypopigmented areas may be more easily appreciated under Wood's
long-wave ultraviolet light.

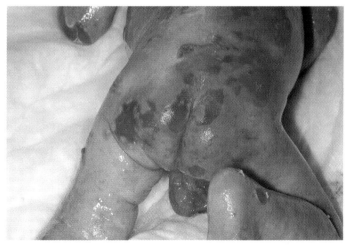

Fig. 17.10 Junctional epidermolysis bullosa
There is extensive fragility of the skin resulting in blistering and subsequent erosions as here. The mucous membranes are involved. The defect
is due to an abnormality of the hemidesmosomes so that the epidermis
does not attach to the dermis properly and is easily disturbed by the
slightest friction and trauma. © Photograph courtesy of Professor Robin
Eady.

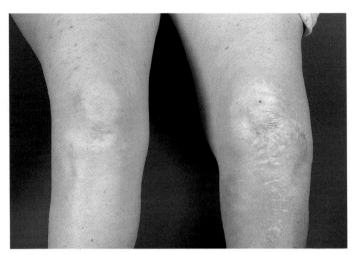

Fig. 17.11 Ehlers–Danlos syndrome
Papyraceous (papery) scars form after minimal injury particularly over pressure points such as the knees and elbows. There are many different types of the disorder but the essential defect is a quantative deficiency of collagen. In some types the joints are hypermobile, which may impair walking. Subluxation of joints, kyphoscoliosis, hernias, varicose veins and premature delivery due to rupture of membranes are all possible complications of the syndrome.

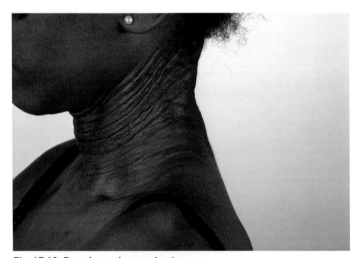

Fig. 17.12 Pseudoxanthoma elasticum
The elastic tissue is abnormal and the skin feels soft, is loose and may hang in folds. The importance of this inherited disorder is that the media and intima of blood vessels, the endocardium and pericardium are involved. Characteristic eye changes known as angioid streaks are visible in the retina as a result of the vascular abnormality.

18 Immunological Disorders

Vitiligo

Definition
A common acquired disorder characterized by destruction of melanocytes by autoantibodies resulting usually in complete loss of pigmentation in the skin, mucous membranes or sometimes the hair.

Characteristics

Symptoms
• loss of pigment
• sometimes a premonitory itch

Signs
• well-defined patches of white skin without any textural change (Fig. 18.1)
• sometimes hypopigmented areas associated with white discoloration in dark-skinned races

Distribution
• anywhere, usually symmetrical
• including circumorificial, intertriginous, genital, acral and on extensor surfaces
• may be extensive and become universal

Variants
• halo naevus
• Koebner phenomenon

Associations
Other autoimmune disorders including thyroid, Addison's, diabetes mellitus and scleroderma.

Differential diagnosis
• pityriasis versicolor
• pityriasis alba
• lichen sclerosus et atrophicus
• piebaldism
• leprosy

Management
- generally poor
- superpotent steroids
- photochemotherapy (PUVA)
- solar protection to reduce contrast with normal skin
- camouflage
- dihydroxyacetone to stain the white skin brown
- monobenzyl ether of hydroquinone to depigment the normal skin
- skin grafts

Alopecia areata

Definition
A loss of hair without appreciable abnormalities of the skin ranging in severity from a localized round patch or patches on the scalp or beard area to a universal abnormality probably due to an autoimmune process. Spontaneous recovery takes place after several months in most limited cases.

Characteristics

Symptoms
A localized patch of hair loss.

Signs
- one or several round patches of hair loss (Fig. 18.2) which may become generalized or universal
- exclamation mark hairs (thin and depigmented hair shaft close to the scalp with normal width of stump) indicate active disease
- the hair is white as it recovers and subsequently repigments

Distribution
- usually all or most of the scalp or beard area
- secondary sex hair may be affected
- in severe cases body hair is shed including eyebrows and eyelashes
- loss of occipital hair (ophiasis) indicates a poor prognosis

Variants
- involvement of the nails especially pitting
- 'going white overnight'

Associations
- other autoimmune disorders including thyroid and vitiligo
- atopic eczema
- Down's syndrome

Differential diagnosis
- tinea capitis
- lupus erythematosus
- traction alopecia
- trichotillomania
- frictional
- of localized disorders of the hair and scalp

Management
- explanation and prognosis (Table 18.1)
- superpotent topical steroids
- intralesional triamcinolone
- photochemotherapy
- minoxidil topically
- immunotherapy

Table 18.1 Factors indicating a less favourable prognosis in alopecia areata

Onset in childhood
Several patches
Ophiasis
Loss of eyebrows and eyelashes
Widespread or universal involvement
Previous atopy
Previous attacks

Bullous pemphigoid

Definition
A serious disorder predominantly affecting the elderly characterized by the spontaneous eruption of itchy large tense blisters due to an autoimmune disorder affecting the dermo-epidermal junction.

Characteristics

Symptoms
Very itchy blisters.

Signs
- large tense bullae containing clear fluid, often surrounded by erythema (Fig. 18.3). They commence as vesicles but rapidly enlarge and subsequently break leaving behind denuded eroded skin often covered with haemorrhagic scabs (Fig. 18.4)
- milia may result as the lesions heal

• sometimes there is a prebullous urticarial stage early on in the evolution of the disease

Distribution
Limbs initially (particularly inner aspects), trunk ultimately.

Complications
Sepsis.

Associations
• other autoimmune disorders
• underlying malignancy (not proven)
• pregnancy (pemphigoid (herpes) gestationis) (Fig. 18.5)

Variants
• benign mucous membrane pemphigoid
• localized bullous pemphigoid

Diagnosis
• clinical
• skin biopsy for histopathology and immunofluorescence (Fig. 18.6)
• blood for circulating antibodies

Differential diagnosis
• insect bites
• pemphigus
• other causes of blistering

Management
• rule out coexistent malignancy
• oral steroids
• other immunosuppressives especially azathioprine for steroid-sparing effect
• antibiotics for sepsis

Pemphigus

Definition
An uncommon but serious autoimmune disorder affecting interepidermal cell cohesion resulting in flaccid blisters and painful erosions of the skin and mucous membranes. It often presents in the mouth. It usually commences in middle age.

Characteristics

Symptoms
A sore mouth or blisters on the body.

Signs
Flaccid bullae (Fig. 18.7) which appear on normal skin and break easily leaving behind painful erosions or crusts. They heal slowly, sometimes with pigmentation, often with scarring.

Distribution
Mucous membrane:
- within the mouth (Fig. 18.8)
- genitalia

Skin, anywhere but especially:
- face
- trunk (Fig. 18.9)
- axillae
- groin
- sometimes in annular configurations

Associations
Other autoimmune processes.

Diagnosis
- clinical
- skin or mucous membrane biopsy for histopathology (Fig. 18.10)
- immunofluorescence
- blood for indirect immunofluorescence
- Tzanck test for acantholysis

Differential diagnosis
Of oral lesions:
- herpes simplex
- hand, foot and mouth disease
- ulcerative lichen planus
- Behçet's syndrome
- benign mucous membrane pemphigoid

Of other genital lesions:
Of skin lesions:
- impetigo
- bullous pemphigoid
- other blistering disorders

Management
- oral steroids

- other immunosuppressives including azathioprine, cyclophosphamide, cyclosporine
- intramuscular gold therapy

Dermatitis herpetiformis

Definition
An extremely itchy disorder associated with a gluten-sensitive but usually asymptomatic enteropathy, resulting in groups of excoriated oedematous papules and vesicles symmetrically distributed in a particular pattern on the elbows, knees, buttocks and scalp and characterized by deposits of IgA in the dermal papillae or along the basement membrane.

Characteristics

Symptoms
A very itchy rash on the elbows, knees and buttocks.

Signs
Groups of excoriated, oedematous, red papules and vesicles (Fig. 18.11).

Distribution
Symmetrically distributed on the extensor surfaces of forearms just below the elbows and shins just below the knees, the buttocks, the fronts and backs of the shoulders and scalp.

Associations
- other autoimmune disorders
- coeliac syndrome but rarely symptomatic
- rarely lymphoma of the bowel

Diagnosis
- clinical
- skin biopsy for histology and immunofluorescence

Differential diagnosis
- scabies
- prurigo
- lichen planus
- other pruritic disorders

Management
- dapsone
- gluten-free diet
- small bowel biopsy rarely indicated

Lupus erythematosus

Definition

A spectrum of disease which may be confined to the skin (discoid lupus erythematosus), be more widespread on the skin with some immunological abnormalities (subacute lupus) or progress to a serious multisystem disorder characterized by high antinuclear and anti-DNA antibodies (systemic lupus).

Characteristics

Symptoms

A rash on the face and sometimes elsewhere.

Signs

Discoid lupus erythematosus (Fig. 18.12)
• well-defined red plaques with an adherent scale and follicular plugging which may result in scarring and post-inflammatory hyperpigmentation

Subacute and systemic lupus erythematosus
• red annular, slightly oedematous plaques
• a livid diffuse blotchy erythema
• vasculitis
• chilblain lupus
• livedo reticularis

Distribution

• light-exposed areas especially the face (cheeks and bridge of nose) and ears but also the V of the neck, front of the chest, backs of hands and arms and elsewhere
• scalp (discoid lupus)
• hair loss (systemic lupus)
• fingers and hands (chilblain lupus)
• around nails

Diagnosis

• clinical
• skin biopsy:
   —for histopathology
   —for immunofluorescence (heavy deposits of several immunoglobulins are found in a band at the basement membrane in non-involved sun-spared skin in systemic lupus)
• autoantibodies.

Differential diagnosis
- facial eruptions (scaly red patches/plaques)
- other photodermatoses

Associations
- arthritis
- serositis
- renal
- central nervous system
- haematological abnormalities:
  —haemolytic anaemia
  —leucopenia
  —lymphopenia
  —thrombocytopenia
- lymphadenopathy
- positive anti-DNA, antismooth muscle and antinuclear antibodies
- false positive serology

Management
Assessment of extent of the disorder.
Varied and specialist based:
- local and systemic steroids
- other immunosuppressives
- hydroxychloroquine and other antimalarials

Dermatomyositis

Definition
An immunological disorder of proximal limb muscle groups causing pain and weakness associated with a characteristic skin eruption affecting especially the eyelids, knuckles and the area around the nails, occurring in both childhood and adult life. The latter variety is sometimes associated with malignancy.

Characteristics

Symptoms
Difficulty in raising the arms above the head and walking upstairs, and a rash.

Signs
- a mauve discoloration (Fig. 18.13)
- purple papules over the knuckles and nail folds (Fig. 18.14)

Distribution
- particularly the upper eyelids with oedema, upper cheeks and temples

- across the backs of the knuckles
- on the back of the neck, elbows and knees
- around the nails (with ragged cuticles)

Associations
- carcinoma of lung, ovary, breast, stomach and cervix or lymphoma in perhaps 25% of adult cases
- Raynaud's phenomenon
- cutaneous calcification

Diagnosis
- clinical
- raised levels of muscle enzymes including creatine phosphokinase
- electromyelogram
- muscle biopsy
- autoantibodies (Jo-1 often positive and antinuclear antibodies sometimes)

Differential diagnosis
Lupus erythematosus.

Management
- exclusion of underlying malignancy in adult cases
- systemic steroids combined with steroid-sparing immunosuppressives such as azathioprine and methotrexate
- rest

Scleroderma (systemic sclerosis)

Definition
A multisystem disorder associated with antinuclear antibodies presenting in the skin initially as Raynaud's phenomenon followed by a gradual tethering of the skin to the subcutaneous tissue affecting the face, hands and feet causing limitation of movement and also necrosis of skin from digital ischaemia.

Characteristics

Symptoms
Fingers go white in the cold; puffy fingers; difficulty straightening the fingers.

Signs
- Raynaud's phenomenon
- tethering and sclerosis of the skin (the skin feels hard, cannot be pinched and the skin creases disappear) causing sausage-like fingers (Fig. 18.15)

initially then tapering of the finger tips due to loss of the finger pulps, a beak-like appearance of the nose and a shrunken mouth with radiating furrows
- matt telangiectases on the face and fingers
- calcinosis of the fingers
- hirsutism
- hyperpigmentation

Distribution
Face, hands and feet.

Associations
- involvement of the gastrointestinal tract (dysphagia and diverticula)
- the lungs (leading to pulmonary fibrosis)
- heart and kidneys

Variants
CREST (calcinosis, Raynaud's, oesophageal involvement, sclerosis and telangiectases).

Diagnosis
- clinical
- autoantibodies (anticentromere antibodies associated with a better prognosis)

Differential diagnosis
- generalized morphoea
- mixed connective tissue disease

Management
Unsatisfactory and varied.

Localized scleroderma (morphoea)

Definition
A localized plaque of sclerosis of the skin without any systemic consequences but often associated with positive autoantibodies.

Characteristics

Symptoms
An abnormal patch of skin.

Signs
A single (sometimes multiple) tethered, sclerotic, shiny, white or mauve plaque of skin (Fig. 18.16) often with a lilac-coloured surround which may ultimately resolve, often leaving a pigmented patch behind.

Distribution
Anywhere but especially the proximal limb or torso.

Variants
* coup de sabre
* generalized morphoea (rare)

Diagnosis
* clinical
* skin biopsy

Differential diagnosis
Lichen sclerosus et atrophicus (Figs 18.17 and 18.4).

Management
Superpotent topical steroids in active stage.

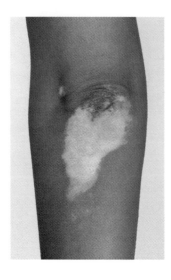

Fig. 18.1 Vitiligo
There is total absence of pigment in a well-defined patch. There is no surface or textural change in the skin. The contrast between normal and abnormal skin is most marked in darker skins. The melanocytes are destroyed by autoantibodies.

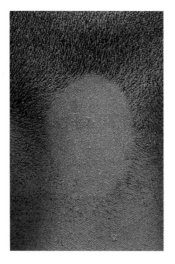

Fig. 18.2 Alopecia areata
There is an almost circular patch of complete loss of hair without any change in the surface or texture of the skin. The prognosis for recovery for a single patch is excellent in an adult with or without treatment. It usually takes 9 months on the scalp but up to 2 years in the beard.

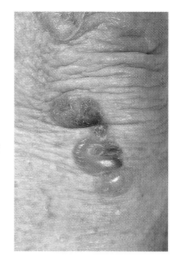

Fig. 18.3 Bullous pemphigoid
The blisters are formed as a result of damage caused by immunoglobulin deposition at the basement membrane, which separates the epidermis from the dermis resulting in the spontaneous appearance of tense firm itchy blisters. There may be a surrounding erythema or oedema.

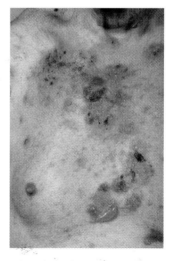

Fig. 18.4 Bullous pemphigoid
The blistering, erosions and haemorrhagic scabs eventually become widespread and the patient requires treatment with prednisolone (usually starting at 40 mg daily) and a steroid-sparing immunosuppressive such as azathioprine.

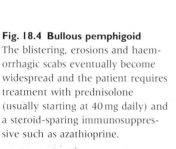

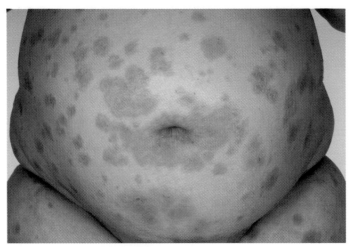

Fig. 18.5 Pemphigoid (herpes) gestationis
This is a very rare disorder occurring at any stage of pregnancy and in all subsequent pregnancies (but not necessarily if there is a change of father). Immunologically it is similar to bullous pemphigoid. It is treated with systemic steroids and remits with parturition.

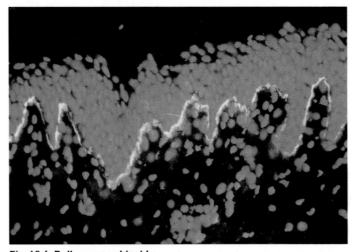

Fig. 18.6 Bullous pemphigoid
There is a yellow band of immunofluorescence due to deposition of IgG at the basement membrane. Bullous pemphigoid is an autoimmune disorder characterized by circulating antibodies to basement membrane between the epidermis and the dermis. © Photograph courtesy of Mr B. Bhogal.

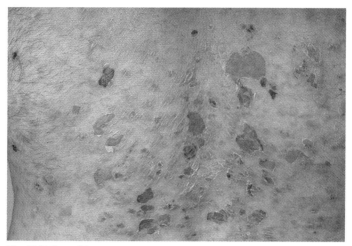

Fig. 18.7 Pemphigus
The blisters are flaccid and break easily leaving raw painful erosions and haemorrhagic crusts which do not heal without treatment.

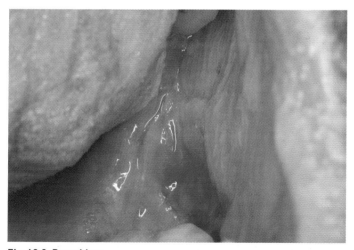

Fig. 18.8 Pemphigus
Pemphigus frequently commences in the mouth with painful erosions which fail to heal. The preceding blisters are usually not visible since they are readily traumatized and break. The diagnosis may be made by biopsy for pathology and immunofluorescence. Pemphigoid is unusual in the mouth except in the benign mucous membrane variety and when pemphigoid is associated with malignancy.

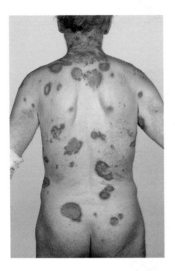

Fig. 18.9 Pemphigus
The blistering takes place within the epidermis so that the roof of the blister is composed of a thinner layer of epidermal cells than in pemphigoid where the roof is made of the entire epidermis. It is for this reason that the blister is flaccid and more fragile than that of pemphigoid. The cells separate away from each other, an appearance known as acantholysis.

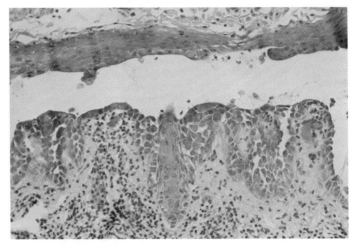

Fig. 18.10 Pemphigus
Pemphigus gradually extends. The condition is painful. The lesions become infected and the patient debilitated. The disorder was likely to be fatal before the advent of systemic steroids. It requires high dosages (80–120 mg prednisolone) compared with other immunosuppressives including azathioprine, cyclophosphamide or gold to induce remission. It is rare but particularly affects Jews.

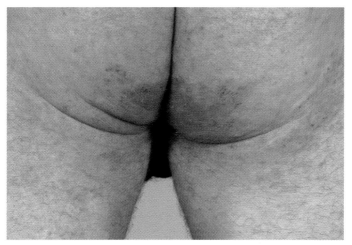

Fig. 18.11 Dermatitis herpetiformis
The eruption is symmetrical and has a particular predilection for certain
sites which are the buttocks, just below the knees and elbows, the back
of the shoulders and the scalp. The condition is more common in those
of Irish ancestry, especially those coming from the west coast. All have
an associated gluten-sensitive enteropathy although rarely symptoms of
coeliac syndrome.

Fig. 18.12 Discoid lupus
erythematosus
There are two well-defined annular
red plaques with an adherent scale
on the cheeks. They are persistent.
The disorder is more common in
females.

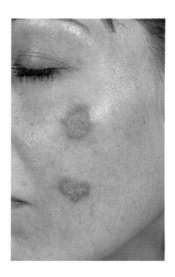

219

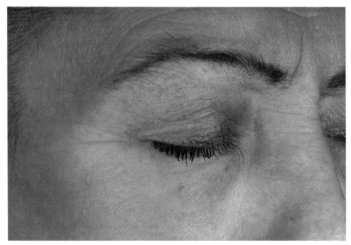

Fig. 18.13 Dermatomyositis
The diagnosis may be made by the colour changes and distribution of the rash over the knuckles and around the eyes. It is associated with discomfort in the proximal limb muscles and thus difficulty in raising the arms above the head and climbing stairs. The muscle enzymes, creatine phosphokinase and the adult variety may be associated with malignancy. Transaminases are raised.

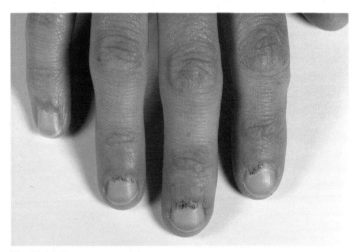

Fig. 18.14 Dermatomyositis
There is a mauve papular eruption (Gottron's papules) over the knuckles. The cuticles are conspicious with haemorrhages in them, a sign which may also occur in lupus erythematosus. The ANF may be positive in the autoimmune variety.

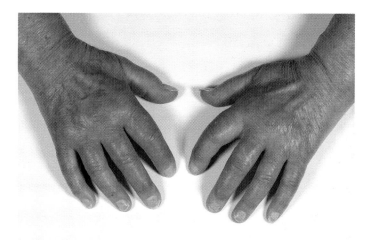

Fig. 18.15 Scleroderma
Patients invariably experience Raynaud's phenomenon initially and the fingers become sausage-shaped. The skin creases are obliterated and the skin is difficult to pinch between the examining fingers and appears shiny.

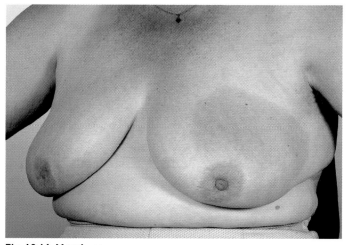

Fig. 18.16 Morphoea
There is a single mauve plaque. The skin usually still feels indurated and tethered at this stage but it does slowly recover although post-inflamatory pigmentation may be long lasting. The breast and abdomen are common sites. The condition, although having the same clinical and histological appearances as scleroderma, has no systemic complications.

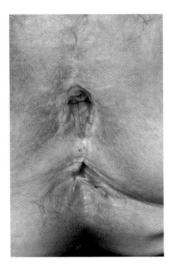

Fig. 18.17 Lichen sclerosis et atrophicus
The white shiny skin can be seen with tethering and distortion of the architecture of the perineum. The condition may be very itchy but is controllable with superpotent steroids. This woman had had an unnecessary vulvectomy, the white areas being accepted clinically as leukoplakia and equated with carcinoma *in situ*. If the clinical diagnosis is in doubt, a biopsy will distinguish the two.

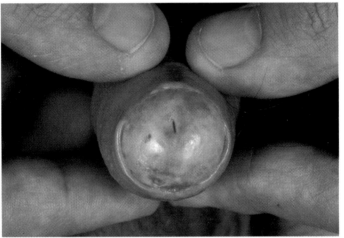

Fig. 18.18 Lichen sclerosus et atrophicus
The patient has difficulty retracting the foreskin. The ivory-white sclerotic shiny skin is apparent on the glans penis with narrowing of the urethral meatus. Haemorrhage in the atrophic skin is visible. Occasionally similar plaques may occur on the skin.

19 Reactive and Drug Eruptions

Urticaria and angio-oedema

Definition

A condition of transient itchy pink swellings of the skin and mucous membranes of various sizes and shapes due to release of histamine and other vasoactive amines from mast cells triggered by a variety of physical and immunological stimuli, occasionally resulting in anaphylaxis and circulatory collapse.

Characteristics

Symptoms

Hives, nettle rash or itchy swellings (sometimes described as blisters).

Signs

- pink or red weals with central pallor (Fig. 19.1)
- dermographism (Fig. 19.2)
- angio-oedema

Distribution

Anywhere including lips, eyelids, hands, genitalia, tongue and larynx (with attendant risk of asphyxia) and anaphylaxis.

Differential diagnosis

- urticarial vasculitis
- other itchy conditions

Management

- identify cause if possible
- antihistamines
- occasionally systemic steroids
- of anaphylaxis—adrenaline, securing airway, etc.

Causes

See Table 19.1.

Toxic erythema

Definition

A generalized red macular or maculopapular (morbilliform) eruption of

Table 19.1 Causes of urticaria

Drugs	*Infection*
IgE mediated:	Viral hepatitis
penicillin	*Candida*
cephalosporins	Protozoa
aspirin	Bacteria
toxoids	
sera	*Immunological disorders*
quinine	Serum sickness
Direct mast cell degranulation:	lymphoma
morphine	Systemic lupus erythematosus
codeine	Macroglobulinaemia
	Polycythaemia
Foods	
Shellfish	*Physical*
Nuts	Dermographism
Eggs	Pressure
Strawberries	Ultraviolet irradiation, cold, heat
Tomatoes	Water (aquagenic)
Pork	Cholinergic
Food additives and dyes	
	Chronic non-allergic
	Atopics

the skin, usually caused by a drug or a virus (often not identified), but not always explicable.

Characteristics

Symptoms
An itchy rash.

Signs
• red macules which may become papular and confluent, looking like a blotchy erythema (morbilliform)
• may subsequently desquamate

Distribution
Widespread; may become universal (erythrodermic) (Fig. 19.3).

Associations
• infectious mononucleosis
• leukaemia

Diagnosis

History of drug ingestion (usually broad-spectrum antibiotic) up to 2 weeks previously.

Differential diagnosis

• viral exanthems
• bacterial exotoxins (e.g. streptococcal erythrotoxin or staphylococcal toxic shock syndrome)
• other truncal eruptions presenting acutely

Management

• identify and stop drug
• calamine
• antihistamines
• occasionally systemic steroids

Erythema nodosum

Definition

An acute outbreak of crops of tender red nodules over the lower legs particularly the shins, occurring as a reaction, probably immune-complex mediated, to a variety of possible causes.

Characteristics

Symptoms

Painful lumps on the legs.

Signs

Red, tender, smooth-surfaced nodules (Fig. 19.4).

Distribution

• fronts of shins
• backs of calves (often tuberculosis)

Variants

Nodular vasculitis.

Diagnosis

• clinical
• skin biopsy

Differential diagnosis

Other eruptions on the shins.

Management

Investigate and treat the cause.

Erythema multiforme

Definition

An acute self-limiting mucocutaneous eruption with a characteristic morphology usually precipitated by a virus, particularly herpes simplex, but occasionally more severe and involving mucous membranes and other organs (Stevens–Johnson syndrome) due to a drug or other noxious agent.

Characteristics

Symptoms

A rash particularly on the extremities often following (on direct questioning) a cold sore.

Signs

Target lesions: round red or purple plaques with a central 'bull's eye' which may be a purple papule (iris type) or vesicle or bulla (vesiculobullous type).

Distribution

• symmetrical particularly on extremities including hands (Fig. 19.5) and feet and genitalia
• sometimes mouth ulceration (Fig. 19.6)

Variants

• Stevens–Johnson syndrome (Fig. 19.7)
• toxic epidermal necrolysis
• recurrent erythema multiforme

Diagnosis

• clinical
• histopathology
• search for the cause

Differential diagnosis

Of iris type:
• unmistakable (Fig. 19.8)
Of bullous type:
• bullous pemphigoid
• other blistering disorders
Of Stevens–Johnson and toxic epidermal necrolysis:
• staphylococcal scalded skin syndrome

Management

Simple erythema multiforme:
• symptomatic
• prophylactic treatment of herpes simplex with acyclovir if recurrent, sometimes long-term immunosuppression with azathioprine
Severe forms:
• hospitalization
• intensive care
• systemic steroids (controversial)

Phototoxic drug eruptions

Definition

An erythema, oedema and sometimes eczema of ultraviolet-light-exposed areas of the skin and/or nails due to the interaction of a drug and sunlight.

Characteristics

Symptoms
A rash on the face and hands and sometimes the V of the neck and the legs.

Signs
Sharply defined redness and sometimes oedema and scaling.

Distribution
Light-exposed areas especially:
• face (except where protected by hair and under nose and chin)
• backs of hands and sometimes forearms
• lower limbs (especially in those who wear skirts or shorts)
• V of neck
• back of neck (sharply defined by collar)

Variants
Photo-onycholysis (Fig. 19.9).

Diagnosis
• clinical
• search for causes (Table 19.2)

Differential diagnosis
Other photodermatoses (Table 19.3) including:
• polymorphic light eruption
• chronic actinic dermatosis (Fig. 19.10)

Table 19.2 Common photosensitizing drugs

Psychotropics
Phenothiazines, especially chlorpromazine and promethazine
Diazepam
Protryptiline
Carbamazepine

Antibiotics
Sulphonamides
Tetracyclines, especially demethylchlortetracycline and vibramycin

Diuretics
Thiazides
Nalidixic acid
Frusemide

Non-steroidal inflammatories
Piroxicam
Naproxen
Feldene

Cardiac
Amiodarone
Atenolol
Propanolol

Diabetic
Chlorpropramide

Dermatological
Griseofulvin
Psoralens

Topical
Tetrachlorsalicylanide in soaps and other toiletries
Psoralens
Promethazine

Management
Identify and withdraw offending drug.

Side-effects of topical steroids
- Acne
  —perioral and periorbital dermatitis
  —monomorphic papulopustular acne

Table 19.3 Classification of photodermatoses

Metabolic diseases	*Degenerative*
Porphyria	Photo-ageing
Xeroderma pigmentosum	
Pellagra	*Pigmentary*
	Melasma
Topical and systemic agents	Pityriasis alba
Phytophotodermatitis	Freckles, lentigines
Drugs	Malignant melanoma
Immunological	*Epidermal*
Solar urticaria	Basal cell papillomas
Polymorphic light eruption	Basal and squamous cell carcinoma
Chronic actinic dermatitis	
Lupus erythematosus	*Disorders affected by sunlight*
	Herpes simplex
	Pityriasis versicolor

- Rosacea
- Folliculitis
- Atrophy of the epidermis and dermis (Fig. 19.11)
  - —telangiectasia
  - —wrinkling
  - —purpura
  - —striae
- Atrophy of the subcutis and loss of pigment
- Immunosuppression (due to misuse)
  - —tinea incognito
  - —pityriasis versicolor
  - —mollusca contagiosa
  - —warts especially plane
  - —scabies
- Generalized pustular psoriasis
- Contact dermatitis
- Adrenal suppression (Fig. 19.12)

Drug eruptions simulating skin disorders
- acneiform, e.g. isoniazid, steroids
- psoriasiform, e.g. β-blockers
- eczematous, e.g. contact dermatitis
- pityriasis rosea-like, e.g. gold
- lichenoid, e.g. gold, antimalarials
- ichthyotic, e.g. carbamazepine

Fixed drug eruption

Definition
The occurrence of a red–brown round swelling which subsides leaving a distinctive round post-inflammatory area of hyperpigmentation and then recurs in the same site each time the noxious agent (often phenolphthalein) is ingested.

Characteristics

Symptoms
Round black marks on the skin (Fig. 19.13).

Signs
Red–brown round oedematous swellings resulting in post-inflammatory pigmentation.

Distribution
Anywhere but especially face, backs of hands, genitalia, limbs or within the mouth.

Differential diagnosis
None necessary.

Management
Identification and withdrawal of the agent.

Causes
- phenolphthalein and other laxatives
- phenacetin
- griseofulvin
- tetracyclines
- sulphonamides

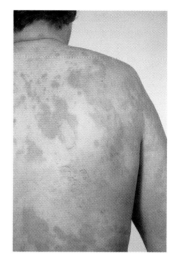

Fig. 19.1 Urticaria
The weals may be widespread. The commonest known causes are drugs such as penicillin and aspirin and foods such as nuts, eggs and shellfish. However, in chronic cases the cause may not be apparent and the condition has to be controlled with prophylactic long-term antihistamines until it goes into spontaneous remission.

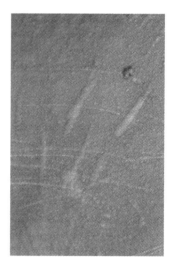

Fig. 19.2 Dermographism
This literally means that one can write on the skin. Thus scratching the skin results in a weal and flare reaction (Lewis' triple response) as seen here. It may occur as an entity in its own right or as part of other urticarial manifestations. The former is particularly common in the young and may persist for months or some years before resolving. Antihistamines are only partially effective at suppressing the reaction.

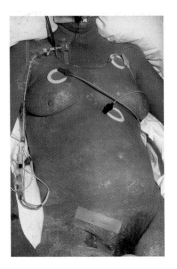

Fig. 19.3 Erythroderma
If a suspected drug is not stopped early and sometimes even if it is, the eruption becomes universal resulting in thermoregulatory abnormalities due to vasodilatation (the patient is often shivering even in a warm room) and haemodynamic abnormalities due to a 5–10 times increase in skin blood flow, which may lead to heart failure.

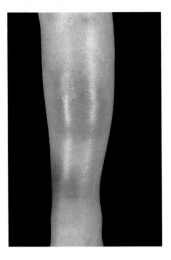

Fig. 19.4 Erythema nodosum
The common causes of these tender red nodules are sarcoidosis, drugs and streptococci. Tuberculosis and leprosy are common worldwide and rarely the condition occurs with lymphoma and inflammatory bowel disease.

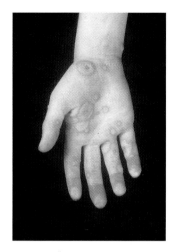

Fig. 19.5 Erythema multiforme
The target lesion is unique to this
condition. It consists of round red
or somewhat purple plaques with a
central ring or 'bull's eye' which
may be a papule or vesicle.

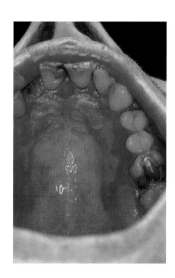

Fig. 19.6 Erythema multiforme
There is denudation of the oral and
genital mucosa secondary to the
epidermal necrosis in more severe
forms. This young man developed
his reaction to herpes simplex, the
commonest cause.

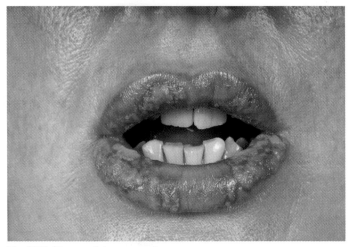

Fig. 19.7 Stevens–Johnson syndrome
Erosions, crusting and ulceration of the mucous membranes, particularly the mouth and lips but also the genitalia, may accompany simple erythema multiforme but are more common with the severe Stevens–Johnson form.

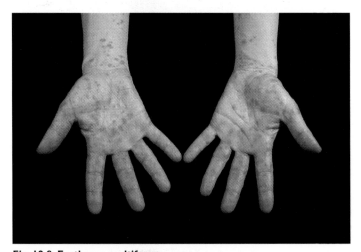

Fig. 19.8 Erythema multiforme
The onset is acute. The lesions are 'multiform' being predominantly red and swollen papules and plaques occurring on the limbs, but the hallmark of the eruption is the target lesion occurring most clearly on the acral areas such as the palms and backs of hands.

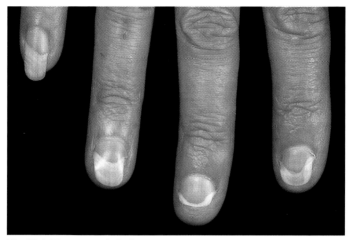

Fig. 19.9 Photo-onycholysis
All the finger- (and sometimes toe-) nails are affected due to an interaction between a drug (often tetracycline) and the sun.

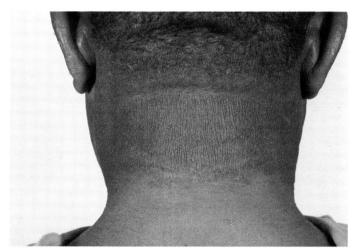

Fig. 19.10 Chronic actinic dermatitis
This is an uncommon persistent eczematous disorder of the summer months usually of elderly males and in which no drug cause is identified. Phototesting shows the patient to be allergic to UVA and sometimes UVB or both. The histology may ultimately be lymphomatous (it was originally called actinic reticuloid) but it has a benign course and does respond to photoprotection and azathioprine (for severe cases). The clue to the diagnosis is the sharp cut off (for example here on the neck) where the clothing has protected the skin.

235

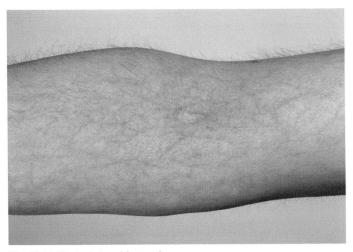

Fig. 19.11 Topical steroid atrophy
There is thinning of the skin with clearly visible dilatation of blood vessels (telangiectasia) due to destruction of collagen. The flexural areas are most vulnerable and long-term use of topical steroids should not be prescribed without regular supervision.

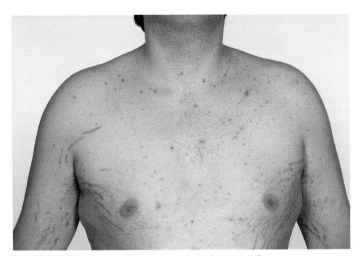

Fig. 19.12 Topical steroid induced adrenal suppression
There are widespread striae. This patient was using 100g of a superpotent steroid every week to treat psoriasis (evidence of which is still present). His plasma cortisol response to synacthen stimulation was severely reduced. Superpotent topical steroids are an unwise long-term treatment for psoriasis.

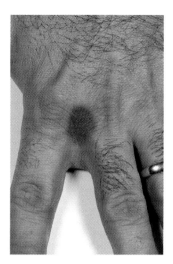

Fig. 19.13 Fixed drug eruption
The condition may become quite extensive. It is often difficult to persuade some patients that it is due to a drug or it may be difficult to identify what agent it is that they are taking. However, stopping the drug does resolve the problem.

20 Vascular and Lymphatic Disorders

Purpura

Definition
Purpura is a physical sign, not a diagnosis. It results from leakage of red blood cells out of vessels thus staining the skin a purple colour which does not blanch on pressure and fades through various colour changes as haem is broken down. Small lesions are known as petechiae and large ones as ecchymoses or bruises. There are many causes but purpura is essentially due to platelet, coagulation or vascular abnormalities. The former are usually non-palpable. Vasculitic or embolic purpura are palpable.

Characteristics

Symptoms
An asymptomatic rash on the lower limbs (purpura/vasculitis) or 'blood spots' (ecchymoses).

Signs
Non-palpable purpura:
• petechiae—small purple macules which do not blanch on pressure (Fig. 20.1)
• ecchymoses—large purple patches which do not blanch on pressure (Fig. 20.2)
Palpable purpura:
• purple papules
• vesiculopustules

Distribution
Anywhere but particularly limbs and buttocks.

Diagnosis
• clinical
• skin biopsy
• search for cause (see Table 20.1)

Allergic vasculitis

Definition
A form of vasculitis characterized in the skin by an infiltration of the small

Table 20.1 Causes of purpura

BLOOD DISORDERS

Platelet abnormalities
Idiopathic thrombocytopenic purpura
Secondary thrombocytopenic purpura
  Bone marrow infiltration (leukaemia, myeloma, carcinomatosis, myelofibrosis)
  Bone marrow arrest or dysfunction (drugs, irradiation, pernicious anaemia)
  Excessive consumption or destruction (e.g. *disseminated intravascular coagulation*, splenomegaly)
  Infections (e.g. septicaemia, typhoid, tuberculosis, hepatitis and other viruses)
  Abnormal platelet function

Coagulation abnormalities
e.g. haemophilia, von Villebrand's disease, protein C or S deficiency

Plasma protein abnormalities
Macroglobulinaemia
Cryoglobulinaemia

BLOOD VESSEL ABNORMALITIES

Defects of vessel walls
  Congenital, e.g. Ehlers–Danlos syndrome, pseudoxanthoma elasticum
  Acquired, e.g. amyloid
Decreased vascular support
  e.g. solar or steroid purpura, scurvy
Damage to blood vessels
  e.g. vasculitis or emboli
Toxic
  e.g. chemicals, drugs, infections
Systemic disease
  e.g. renal, liver disease, diabetes and carcinomatosis
Raised intravascular pressure
  e.g. stasis
Capillaritis
  e.g. pigmented purpuric eruption

---

blood vessels of the upper dermis by neutrophils which release their nuclei as debris (or 'dust'). There is extravasation of red cells and fibrinoid necrosis (a mixture of fibrin degradation products) in the vessel walls. This characteristic histological picture is known as a leucocytoclastic vasculitis and may represent an immune-complex disorder. Other organs, particularly the kidneys, may be affected. Infections, drugs, lupus erythematosus and malignancy may cause it but often the cause is obscure. A similar condition occurring mainly in young boys is known as Henoch–Schönlein purpura.

Characteristics

Symptoms
Acute rash on the lower limbs and buttocks, it may be uncomfortable.

Signs
Purpuric macules, papules, vesicles, wheals and bullae resulting in necrosis and sometimes ulceration occurring in crops usually over several weeks.

Distribution
- ankles
- legs (Fig. 20.3)
- buttocks
- occasionally arms

Associations
May be preceded by upper respiratory tract infection and accompanied by arthralgia and mild constitutional upset.

Variants
Henoch–Schönlein (anaphylactoid) purpura (Fig. 20.4).

Diagnosis
- clinical
- skin biopsy
- immunofluorescence for deposits of IgA in the skin

Differential diagnosis
- other causes of vasculitis
- other disorders affecting the lower limbs

Management
Investigations to determine whether other organs (particularly renal) are involved. Treatment includes systemic steroids.
   If cutaneous only:
- symptomatic treatment
- occasionally systemic steroids or dapsone

Pityriasis lichenoides

Definition
A benign disorder of unknown aetiology but characterized by an infiltrate of lymphocytes in and around small blood vessels. It is probably immune-complex mediated and manifests itself in two forms: a chronic erythematosquamous papular eruption on the limbs; and a more acute variety with a purpuric varicelliform morphology and sometimes mild constitutional upset. Both variants may coexist.

Pityriasis lichenoides chronica

Characteristics

Symptoms
A rash on the limbs.

Signs
Many papules at different stages of evolution. They commence as a purple macule which rapidly becomes a red–brown papule, which as it flattens becomes pink with an adherent scale.

Distribution
Scattered mainly over the limbs, particularly the inner aspects (Fig. 20.5), but may occur on the trunk.

Pityriasis lichenoides acuta et varioliformis

Characteristics

Symptoms
An abrupt onset of a rash which is often misdiagnosed as chickenpox.

Signs
A polymorphic eruption of oedematous, often purpuric, papules or vesiculopustules which develop a crust which may eventually become a varioliform scar (Fig. 20.7).

Distribution
Limbs and trunk and occasionally acral areas.

Variants
Lymphomatoid papulosis.

Associations
Occasionally lymphoma.

Diagnosis
• clinical
• biopsy for histopathology

Differential diagnosis
Of pityriasis lichenoides chronica:
• guttate psoriasis
• secondary syphilis
• lichen planus
• mycosis fungoides

Table 20.2 Causes of vasculitis

Small blood vessels
Polymorphonuclear cell infiltration
   Allergic vasculitis
   Henoch–Schönlein syndrome
   Drugs (hypersensitivity angiitis)
   Connective tissue disorders
   Pyoderma gangrenosum
   Behçet's syndrome
   Urticarial vasculitis with hypocomplementaemia

Lymphocytic infiltration
   Drugs
   Erythema multiforme
   Pityriasis lichenoides
   Dysproteinaemias

Granulomatous
   Wegener's granulomatosis
   Lymphomatoid
   Churg–Strauss allergic granulomatosis

Large blood vessels
Polymorphonuclear
   Polyarteritis nodosa
   Superficial migratory thrombophlebitis

Lymphocytic
   Peripheral vascular disease
   Lupus erythematosus

Granulomatous
   Giant cell arteritis (temporal arteritis and polymyalgia rheumatica)
   Takayasu's syndrome

- papular acrodermatitis of childhood

Of pityriasis lichenoides acuta et varioliformis:
- chickenpox
- allergic vasculitis

Management
- phototherapy
- various other treatments including antibiotics and dapsone

Varicose insufficiency, eczema and ulceration

Definition
A common disorder of the skin of the lower extremities due to venous

hypertension secondary to venous thrombosis, genetic absence of the venous valves or a compromised muscle pump resulting in eczema and/or ulceration of the skin.

Characteristics

Symptoms
An itchy rash on the legs or leg ulcer.

Signs
Pigmentation
A patchy macular pigmentation due to haemosiderin deposition secondary to extravasation of red blood cells (petechiae may also be seen) and post-inflammatory melanin deposition

Eczema
• ill-defined, red scaling patches often round, excoriated and in close approximation to the varicosities (Fig. 2.17)
• acute red and vesicular (dermatitis medicamentosa)

Venous flare
Tortuous dilated veins around the ankles

Varicosities and thread veins

Oedema

Cellulitis
A red painful and tender inflammation often around the varicosities

Lipodermatosclerosis
A fibrosis resulting from repeated infection (cellulitis) which produces an indurated sclerodermatous appearance of the lower third of the leg. The contrast between the tapered fibrotic lower third and the swollen upper two thirds makes the leg look like an inverted champagne bottle

Atrophie blanche
White sclerotic macules with red stippling of their surface resulting from necrosis of the skin often following thrombosis in the iliac veins or inferior vena cava

Ulceration
There is a complete break in the epithelium due to the failure of cutaneous nutrition. The ulcer(s) is well defined and the edge is not raised. The base of the ulcer varies from red and haemorrhagic (indicating vascularity and a reasonable chance of healing) to oozing pus (indicating sepsis) and dry, yellow and avascular

Distribution
• lower legs
• and ulcers particularly around the malleoli (Fig. 20.6)

Table 20.3 Clinical distinction between the skin and ulcers of venous and arterial disease

	Venous	Arterial
Ulcers	Usually no discomfort around malleoli	Painful Occur on shins, toes and heels
Skin	Eczema and pigmentation Hair present Normal nails	Dry, atrophic scaly, shiny skin Hair absent Dystrophic nails
Circulation	Pulses present Warm peripheries No cyanosis	Pulses diminished or absent Cool peripheries Cyanotic, purple or blotchy erythema

Differential diagnosis

Of varicose eczema:
• eruptions on lower legs
Of ulcers on the lower limbs:
• infection:
   —deep mycoses
   —gumma
   —lupus vulgaris
   —leprosy
• genetic:
   —Klinefelter's syndrome
   —sickle cell/thalassaemia
• neoplasia:
   —basal cell carcinoma
   —squamous cell carcinoma
   —malignant melanoma
• vascular:
   —pyoderma gangrenosum (Fig. 21.1)
   —necrobiosis lipoidica (Fig. 21.12)
   —vasculitis
   —erythema induratum
   —venous (stasis, postphlebitic)
   —arterial
• neurological
• trauma

Management of venous insufficiency

• avoidance of prolonged standing
• elevation of the leg at rest
• compression bandages to limit oedema

- exercise to utilize the calf muscle pump
- reduction of weight
- diagnosis and treatment of other general medical problems (e.g. anaemia, hypertension, heart failure)
- investigation (patch tests) and treatment of eczema
- treatment of any infection
- local cleaning agents
- surgical management of varicosities and perforators
- skin grafts for ulcers

Arterial leg ulcers

Definition
Cutaneous malnutrition due to arterial insufficiency leading to ulceration of the skin.

Characteristics

Symptoms
Leg ulcer(s), often painful.

Signs
A punched-out quite deep ulcer with a thick necrotic slough associated with poor or absent peripheral pulses.

Signs of cutaneous malnutrition, which are:
- sparse or absent hair on the lower legs and feet
- thickened distorted toe nails, which require cutting less frequently and may be infected with tinea
- dry scaly and atrophic skin
- skin cool to touch
- pale, cyanosed or blotchy livid colour
- gangrene

Distribution
Lower legs and feet (Fig. 20.8).

Associations
- atherosclerosis
- hypertension
- diabetes mellitus
- smoking

Diagnosis
- clinical
- examination of peripheral pulses
- Doppler ultrasound techniques

Differential diagnosis
- venous ulceration
- other causes of leg ulcers

Management
- referral to a vascular surgeon
- control of any associated contributory factors (weight, diabetes, smoking, hypertension)
- cleaning of ulcer(s) but less effective than for venous ulceration

Perniosis (chilblains)

Definition
Localized painful or itchy inflammatory papules of the fingers and toes induced by abnormally prolonged vasoconstriction, resulting in a localized vasculitis followed by a reactive hyperaemia in response to cold climatic conditions.

Characteristics

Symptoms
Itchy spots on the fingers and toes in cold weather which are often painful on rewarming.

Signs
Crops of dusky red or purple slight oedematous papules.

Distribution
Fingers and toes.

Differential diagnosis
- lupus erythematosus (chilblain lupus)
- cutaneous infarcts due to emboli (Fig. 20.9)

Management
- measures to ensure a warm environment
- ultraviolet light
- nifedipine

Raynaud's phenomenon

Definition
A painful paroxysmal condition of the fingers and toes induced by cold which manifests as pallor and coolness followed by cyanosis and subsequently a reactive hyperaemia.

Characteristics

Symptoms
Fingers (and sometimes toes) that go white, blue and red in cold weather and may be painful.

Signs and distribution
Often none at the time of presentation in a warm consulting room but colour changes may be induced by cold.

Causes
- collagen vascular disorders, especially scleroderma and mixed connective tissue disease
- cryoglobulinaemia and cold agglutinins
- compression of the sympathetic nervous system, e.g. cervical rib
- occlusive arterial disease, e.g. Buerger's disease
- toxins:
  —ergotism
  —heavy metals
  —vinyl chloride
- occupational, e.g. pneumatic drills
- smoking
- idiopathic

Management
- of underlying condition if present
- common-sense measures to improve warmth and avoid precipitating conditions in the idiopathic type
- nifedipine
- intra-arterial infusion of various agents including reserpine, prostaglandin E, prostacyclin and low-molecular-weight dextran
- sympathectomy

Livedo reticularis

Definition
This is a physical sign of a dusky erythema occurring in a net-like pattern on the limbs due to a disorder of the blood vessels in the superficial plexus of the dermis.

Characteristics

Symptoms
A rash on the limbs.

Signs
A reticulate erythema (Fig. 20.10).

Distribution
Upper and lower limbs.

Causes
Inflammation of vessel wall:
- idiopathic
- polyarteritis nodosa
- connective tissue disorders
- Sneddon's syndrome (lupus anticoagulant)
- bacterial endocarditis
- syphilis
- TB
- arteriosclerosis and hypertension
- thromboangiitis obliterans
- pancreatitis
- erythema ab igne

Vascular occlusion:
- Arterial embolism
- thrombocythemia
- cryoglobulinaemia
- intravascular coagulation
- cerebrovascular diseases

Diagnosis
- clinical
- skin biopsy

Management
Treatment of the cause.

Lymphoedema

Definition
An initially pitting but subsequently non-pitting oedema of the lower limbs resulting either from a congenital, often inherited, hypoplasia of lymphatics or as a sequel to lymphatic obstruction. Isolated lymphoedema of the lip, eyelids or genitalia may occur.

Characteristics

Symptoms
A localized area of swelling.

Signs and distribution
Oedema (usually non-pitting) of one or both limbs with elephantiasis (a warty hyperkeratosis) in long-standing cases (Fig. 20.11).

Table 20.4 Causes of lower limb lymphoedema

Primary (Milroy's disease)	Congenital (present at birth)
	Praecox (occurring before the age of 35)
	Tarda (occurring after the age of 35)
Secondary	Associated with venous disease
	Immobility (desk chair legs)
	Infection e.g. erysipelas, filariasis
	Neoplastic infiltration e.g. lymphoma, prostatic cancer
	Lymph node block dissection
	Post radiotherapy
	Kaposi's sarcoma

Associations
- ovarian dysgenesis with primary lymphoedema
- lymphangiosarcoma (extremely rare)

Diagnosis
- clinical
- ultrasound (abdominal/pelvic)
- CT scan
- lymphangiography (lower limbs)

Differential diagnosis
- other causes of peripheral oedema (cardiac, renal, hypoalbumenaemia)
- venous insufficiency
- arteriovenous anastomases and other causes of limb hypertrophy

Variants
- oedema of the lower lip (granulomatous cheilitis)
- oedema of the eyelids
- oedema of genitalia

Management
- of the underlying cause
- exercise to increase muscle pump
- elevation and compression with hosiery to move fluid
- massage
- emollients and keratolytics for hyperkeratosis
- long-term penicillin to prevent infection
- surgery

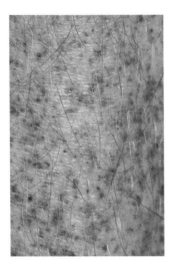

Fig. 20.1 Purpura
There are small purple macules, some of which have gone brown as they fade. The colour cannot be blanched out by pressure over the skin unlike an erythema. This man had thrombocytopenia.

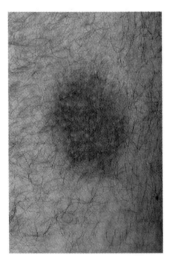

Fig. 20.2 Purpura (ecchymosis)
This man had haemophilia. The large purpuric patch is well illustrated as are the colours that result as haem is broken down within the bruise. The commonest causes of drug-induced bleeding into the skin are anticoagulants which produce large areas of haemorrhage (ecchymoses), or myelosuppressants which produce thrombocytopenia and petechiae.

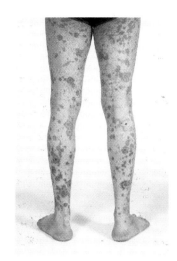

Fig. 20.3 Vasculitis
Drugs may cause vasculitis but not so frequently. The purpura is palpable with papules which may coalesce forming plaques with, in this case, quite annular configurations.

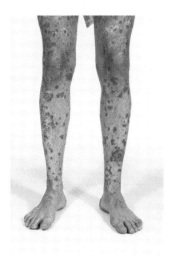

Fig. 20.4 Henoch–Schönlein purpura
This is a syndrome of abdominal pain and sometimes bloody diarrhoea, arthralgia, allergic vasculitis and fever occurring particularly in boys. The condition is self-limiting but there may be associated glomerulonephritis which may require systemic steroids to prevent permanent renal damage. The histology of the rash is of a leucocytoclastic vasculitis and this term, allergic vasculitis, anaphylactoid purpura and Henoch–Schönlein purpura are often used interchangeably.

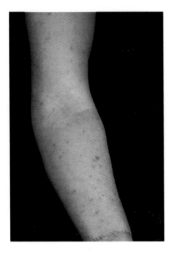

Fig. 20.5 Pityriasis lichenoides chronica
The condition occurs symmetrically particularly on the limbs (especially the inner aspects). It is chronic and difficult to treat although it does respond temporarily to ultraviolet light therapy.

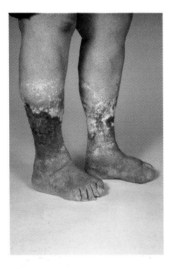

Fig. 20.6 Venous ulceration
There is a complete break in the epithelium secondary to poor cutaneous nutrition. The skin around the malleoli is particularly affected. The ulcer is well defined with a flat margin. The base is red indicating a sufficient blood supply for there to be a reasonable chance of healing—which did occur with simple old-fashioned remedies of gentian violet coupled with potassium permanganate soaks.

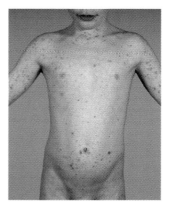 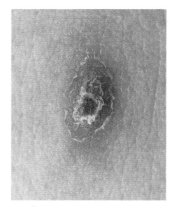

Fig. 20.7 Pityriasis lichenoides acuta

This variety may simply have a more acute onset and subsequently become chronic or disappear after a few weeks. Immune complexes have been demonstrated in the blood vessels but the cause (possibly an infective agent) has not been identified. There may be only a few purpuric oedematous lesions, which are scattered asymmetrically on the body and limbs. There is greater damage to the epidermis than in the chronic variant, sometimes causing blistering and necrosis and hence the title varioliformis (i.e. like chickenpox) for which it may be mistaken.

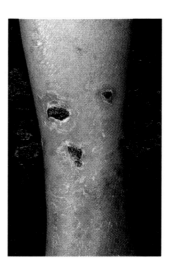

Fig. 20.8 Arterial insufficiency

The results of impaired arterial blood supply of the skin of the lower legs are dryness, loss of hair, atrophy, ulceration often on the shin and painful and cyanotic discoloration of the skin with loss of the peripheral pulses and dystrophy of the toe nails.

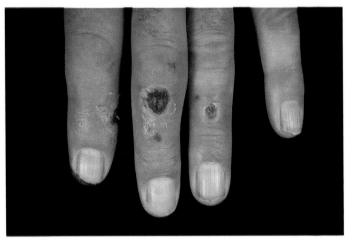

Fig. 20.9 Cutaneous infarcts due to emboli
There are multiple focal areas of necrosis of the skin of the fingers secondary in this case to emboli from an aneurysm of the left ventricle. Other causes include thrombi from valvular disease, endocarditis, atrial fibrillation and myocardial infarction.

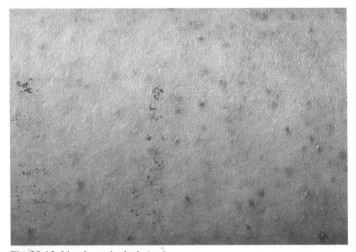

Fig. 20.10 Livedo reticularis
Patients sometimes develop a reticulate (net-like) mauve appearance on their limbs in lupus erythematosus. The differential diagnosis will include antiphospholipid syndrome characterized by anticardiolipin antibodies, recurrent thromboses and miscarriages.

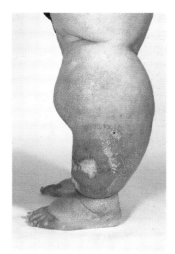

Fig. 20.11 Lymphoedema of the lower limb
There is gross oedema of the lower leg but not of the foot. Some cases are present at birth, most have developed before the age of 35 but some do develop later. Episodes of secondary infection are common and prevented by long-term low doses of penicillin or erythromycin.

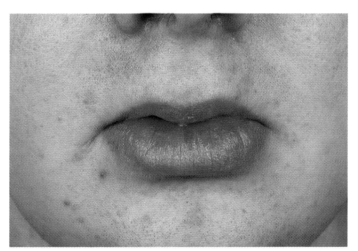

Fig. 20.12 Lymphoedema of the lip (granulomatous cheilitis)
There is lymphoedema of the lower lip. It presents acutely and is occasionally associated with a facial palsy when it is known as the Melkersson–Rosenthal syndrome. it responds partially to injections of triamcinolone under local anaesthesia. The cause is unknown but the pathology is granulomatous and it is sometimes associated with Crohn's disease.

21 Systemic Disorders

INFLAMMATORY DISORDERS

Pyoderma gangrenosum

Definition
An uncommon disorder, which evolves from a sterile pustule or boil-like lesion into an ulcer with a characteristic blue, somewhat oedematous margin. Pathologically it consists of a sterile abscess with a massive infiltrate of neutrophils with haemorrhage and thrombosis and is usually associated with inflammatory bowel disease, rheumatoid arthritis or a blood dyscrasia.

Characteristics

Symptoms
One or several painful ulcers.

Signs
A sterile inflamed pustule or boil which rapidly becomes an ulcer, with a blue or purple oedematous margin (Fig. 21.1). Sterile pustules at sites of trauma, e.g. venepuncture.
Non-cutaneous symptoms and signs:
- fever
- neutrophilia

Distribution
Anywhere but often lower legs.

Causes
Inflammatory:
- rheumatoid arthritis
- Crohn's disease
- ulcerative colitis
- Behçet's syndrome

Haematological:
- plasma cell abnormalities
- monoclonal gammopathies
- hypergammaglobulinaemia
- multiple myeloma
- acute leukaemia
- polycythaemia rubra vera

Cryptogenic:
• but often precipitated by trauma

Diagnosis
• clinical
• histopathology
• microbiology (negative)

Differential diagnosis
• other ulcerative disorders

Management
• of the underlying cause
• systemic steroids, other immunosuppressives (including cyclosporin) and minocycline

Behçet's syndrome

Definition
A triple-symptom complex of recurrent painful ulceration of the mouth and genitalia associated with arthritis and uveitis which may evolve into a life-threatening multisystem disease, which is more common in the Middle East and Japan.

Characteristics

Symptoms
Oral and genital ulceration.

Signs
• oral and genital aphthae
• sterile pustules or pyodermatous lesions especially at sites of injury
• erythema nodosum

Distribution
• ulceration within the mouth, especially the palate (Fig. 21.2)
• ulceration on the genitalia especially the root of the penis, the scrotum and labia
• the pustule or boil-like lesions may occur anywhere but usually at sites of trauma particularly iatrogenic
• erythema nodosum on the lower limbs

Associations
Cutaneous:
• oral/genital ulceration
• pyodermas
• erythema nodosum

Non-cutaneous:
- fever
- arthralgias and large (usually) joint swelling
- iridocyclitis, uveitis, retinal vasculitis, optic atrophy
- neurological abnormalities

Diagnosis
- clinical
- no specific test
- biopsy of skin 48 hours after injection of saline or histamine may show vasculitis

Differential diagnosis
- pemphigus
- other causes of oral/genital ulceration

Management
Nil specific therefore complex (systemic steroids and other immunosuppressives, colchicine).

Sarcoidosis

Definition
A multisystem disorder of unknown aetiology characterized by a non-caseating granulomatous pathology and a positive Kveim test.

Characteristics (cutaneous)

Symptoms
Asymptomatic skin eruption or painful lumps on legs.

Signs
- red–brown smooth-surfaced papules, nodules or plaques (Fig. 21.3)
- purple cyanotic plaques on the nose, cheeks or ear lobes (lupus pernio; Fig. 21.4)
- annular configurations (Fig. 21.5)
- erythema nodosum

Distribution
- trunk, limbs and in black people especially the face (nose and around the eyes) and hands
- invasion of old scars and Mantoux sites
- nose, cheeks, ear lobes (lupus pernio)
- shins (erythema nodosum associated with hilar adenopathy)

Variants
Hypopigmented macules or papules in black people.

Associations

Pulmonary:
• hilar adenopathy, pulmonary infiltrates and fibrosis
Hepatomegaly, lymphadenopathy and splenomegaly
Eyes:
• uveitis
• conjunctivitis
• retinal involvement
• keratoconjunctivitis sicca
Nervous system:
• Bell's palsy
• optic neuritis
• mononeuritis multiplex
• hypothalamic involvement
Cardiac:
• cardiomyopathy
• conduction abnormalities
• heart block
Hypercalcaemia
Bone cysts in terminal phalanges

Diagnosis

• biopsy of the skin or if not involved of other tissue including liver
• Kveim test
• general medical investigations including: serum angiotensin-converting enzyme, calcium studies, and chest and hand X-rays

Differential diagnosis

Other nodular eruptions.

Management

• steroids (intralesional and systemic)
• other immunosuppressives and antimalarials

METABOLIC DISORDERS

Xanthomatosis

Definition

The deposition of lipids in the skin either as a result of an inherited defect of lipoprotein metabolism (the main consequence of which is atheroma and vascular disease) or secondary to a variety of diseases.

Cutaneous characteristics

Symptoms

Yellow spots in the skin.

Signs
- flat yellow plaques around the eyes (xanthelasma; Fig. 21.6)
- yellow papules or nodules

Distribution
- around the eyes (xanthelasma)
- over tendons of elbows, knees, heels and backs of hands
- creases of palms
- eruptive over buttocks, limbs and trunk (Fig. 21.7)

Diagnosis
- clinical
- biopsy rarely necessary
- estimation of major cholesterol fractions and triglycerides
- lipoprotein electrophoresis
- screen family if primary
- search for secondary causes (Table 21.1)

Differential diagnosis
- of xanthelasma—senile milia
- of xanthomata—not usually necessary

Table 21.1 Causes of secondary hyperlipidaemia

Liver disorders
Primary biliary cirrhosis
Haemachromatosis
Congenital atresia or hypotresia
   (Allergele's syndrome) of bile ducts

Renal
Nephrotic syndrome

Pancreatic
Chronic pancreatitis
Diabetes mellitus

Hormonal
Myxoedema

Drugs
Oestrogen
Alcohol abuse
Thiazides

Management
- identification of type if primary and of cause if secondary
- lipid-lowering agents
- dietary manipulation
- superpotent steroids
- Haelan tape
- intralesional triamcinolone

Porphyria cutanea tarda

Definition
The most common of a spectrum of genetically determined enzyme defects in the biosynthesis of haem resulting in the accumulation of precursors, some of which are photosensitizers and others of which give rise to acute neurological, psychiatric and gastrointestinal disturbances. Porphyria cutanea tarda commences in the middle years (tarda) as a photosensitive skin eruption which may be associated with liver damage.

Cutaneous characteristics

Symptoms
Fragile skin and blisters on exposed skin, particularly the backs of the hands.

Signs
- vesicles, blisters or erosions (Fig. 21.8)
- skin that breaks easily
- hypertrichosis
- premature ageing of the skin
- scarring and sclerodermatous changes

Distribution
- sun-exposed areas, especially backs of fingers and hands
- the face

Diagnosis
Estimations of urine, red cell and faecal porphyrins.

Differential diagnosis
- of blistering eruptions
- of photosensitivity

Management

Porphyria cutanea tarda:
- stop alcohol if relevant
- venesection
- chloroquine

Other types:
- complex (specialist referral)

ENDOCRINE DISORDERS

Cutaneous signs and associations

Thyroid disease

Hyperthyroidism:
- Pretibial myxoedema (see section below)
- Vitiligo
- Alopecia areata
- Hair loss
- Palmar erythema
- Onycholysis
- Hyperhidrosis
- Pruritus

Hypothyroidism:
- Myxoedema (Fig. 21.9)
- Ichthyosis
- Hair loss
- Ecchymoses

Diabetes mellitus
- Infection (particularly candidosis)
- Necrobiosis lipoidica (see section below)
- Granuloma annulare (see section below)
- Lichen planus
- Eruptive xanthomatosis
- Secondary to arteriosclerosis

Cutaneous signs and associations of cortisol metabolism

Cushing's disease/syndrome (including topical steroids):
- Atrophy and transparency of the skin with telangiectasia
- Ecchymoses
- Striae (Fig. 21.10)
- Plethoric facies
- Acne
- Hirsutism
- Superficial fungal infections

Addison's disease:
- Increased pigmentation

Pretibial myxoedema

Definition
A localized mucinous infiltration of the dermis producing nodules and plaques on the shins and occasionally feet associated with Graves' disease and elevated serum levels of long-acting thyroid-stimulating hormone.

Characteristics

Symptoms
Patches on the shins (Fig. 21.11).

Signs
Lesions: nodules on a background of a plaque.
Colour: flesh-coloured or pink.
Surface: prominent hair follicle openings; hypertrichosis.
Shape: any but well-defined.

Distribution
Shins.

Diagnosis
• clinical
• skin biopsy

Differential diagnosis
Virtually diagnostic but of any eruption on the shins.

Management
• of associated thyroid disease
• superpotent steroids

Necrobiosis lipoidica

Definition
A degenerative disorder of dermal collagen occurring predominantly on the shins, consisting of well-defined yellowish plaques often of unknown aetiology but associated with diabetes mellitus in half of the patients, which may be due to diabetic micro-angiopathy.

Characteristics

Symptoms
Asymptomatic plaques on the legs.

Signs
Lesions: plaques.
Colour: yellow or red.
Surface: smooth with a waxy consistency; telangiectasia.
Shape: well-defined but varied.

Distribution
Shins (Fig. 21.12), usually bilaterally, occasionally dorsa of feet.

Diagnosis
• clinical
• skin biopsy

Differential diagnosis
Other lesions on the shins.

Management
• glucose tolerance test if indicated
• intralesional triamcinolone (not very helpful)

Granuloma annulare

Definition
A not uncommon disorder of unknown aetiology characterized by red, annular smooth-surfaced plaques with a raised papular margin occurring particularly over the knuckles, elbows, ankles and knees, and a focal destruction of collagen surrounded by a granulomatous response.

Characteristics

Symptoms
Red rings on the skin usually misdiagnosed as ringworm.

Signs
Small, smooth-surfaced firm red or flesh-coloured papules which join together at the rim forming an annular eruption often with a central flattened area.

Distribution
Anywhere, but especially:
• dorsal surfaces of hands
• fingers and feet (Fig. 21.13)
• ankles
• elbows
• knees
May be widespread.

Associations

Family or personal history of diabetes mellitus.

Diagnosis

• clinical
• skin biopsy

Differential diagnosis

• tinea corporis

MALIGNANT DISEASE

Cutaneous signs of malignant disease (paraneoplastic dermatoses)

• generalized pruritus (Table 21.2; Fig. 21.14)
• acquired ichthyosis
• migratory superficial thrombophlebitis
• dermatomyositis
• malignant acanthosis nigricans (Fig. 21.15)
• bullous pemphigoid
• figurate annular erythema
• necrolytic migratory erythema
• Paget's disease of the nipple (see section below)
• extramammary Paget's disease
• mycosis fungoides (see section below)
• Sézary syndrome

Table 21.2 The causes of generalized pruritus

Haematological	*Malignancy*
Iron deficiency anaemia	Lymphoma
Polycythaemia rubra vera	Leukaemia
Paraproteinaemia	Abdominal cancer
Hepatic disease	*Endocrine*
Primary biliary cirrhosis	Hyperthyroidism
Extra hepatic obstruction	Diabetes mellitus
Cholestasis of pregnancy	
Cholestatic drugs	*Idiopathic*
	Prurigo
Renal disease	
Chronic renal failure	*Psychological*
Drugs	
e.g. Morphine	

- localized spread of tumour
- secondary deposits (Fig. 21.16)

Cutaneous Paget's disease

Definition
A skin disorder affecting the nipple associated with an intraductal carcinoma of the breast. It occasionally presents in extramammary sites and is also a sign of underlying regional carcinoma.

Characteristics

Symptoms
A lesion on the nipple.

Signs
A well-defined red scaly or slightly eroded plaque.

Distribution
The nipple (Fig. 21.17).

Diagnosis
Skin biopsy.

Differential diagnosis
- eczema

Variants
Extramammary Paget's disease (anogenital)

Management
Investigation and treatment of underlying carcinoma.

Mycosis fungoides

Definition
An uncommon T-cell lymphoma which presents in the skin and for the most part remains there but which may spread to involve lymph nodes and other organs.

Characteristics

Symptoms
An asymptomatic or sore rash.

Signs
- well-defined pink or red, slightly wrinkled and scaly patches of various sizes and shapes, often rather angulated, plaques and occasionally nodules
- poikiloderma
- may be hypo- or hyperpigmented in black skins

Distribution
Asymmetrical on limbs and trunk (Figs 21.18 and 21.20).

Variants
- digitate dermatosis (chronic superficial scaly dermatosis)
- Sézary syndrome

Associations
Occasionally Hodgkin's and non-Hodgkin's lymphoma.

Diagnosis
- clinical
- biopsy

Differential diagnosis
Mycosis fungoides:
- eczema
- psoriasis
- B-cell lymphoma of the skin

Sézary syndrome (Fig. 21.19):
- other causes of erythroderma
- eczema
- psoriasis
- drug eruptions
- pityriasis rubra pilaris (Fig. 21.21)

Management
Early stages:
- PUVA
- topical nitrogen mustard
- local radiotherapy, electron beam therapy

Late stages:
- various chemotherapeutic regimes

POLYMORPHIC ERUPTION OF PREGNANCY

Pruritic urticarial papules and plaques of pregnancy

Definition

A common, intensely itchy disorder of the last days of the final trimester of the first pregnancy, which disappears immediately after delivery.

Characteristics

Symptoms

Intense itch in pregnancy.

Signs

Urticarial papules and plaques (Fig. 21.22).

Distribution

Commences in the abdominal striae and spreads to the limbs and body.

Differential diagnosis

- other itchy disorders
- other pregnancy eruptions (Table 21.3)

Management

Symptomatic (calamine and antihistamines) but no effective treatment other than delivery.

Table 21.3 The skin and pregnancy

Skin manifestations of the pregnant state
- spider naevi
- palmar erythema
- general pigmentation
- pigmentation of the areola, genitalia and linea alba
- chloasma
- increase in melanocytic naevi
- skin tags
- striae
- increased hair growth
- subsequent telogen effluvium
- pruritus

Skin eruptions occurring during pregnancy
- prurigo gravidarum
- polymorphic eruption of pregnancy
- pemphigoid gestationis

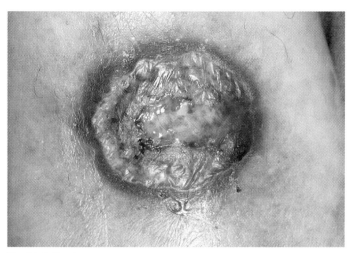

Fig. 21.1 Pyoderma gangrenosum
There is an ulcer with a characteristic purple oedematous and blistering margin. Lesions develop on the shins and elsewhere, particularly at sites of medical intervention, probably as a result of a defective immunological response. It responds to systemic steroids or other immunosuppressives.

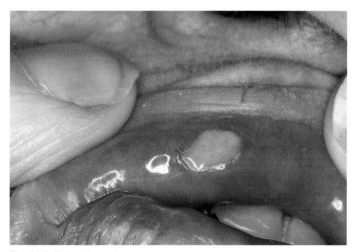

Fig. 21.2 Behçet's syndrome
There is an ulcer with a yellow base similar to a common apthous ulcer, but recurrent lesions also occur on the genitalia, with arthritis and iritis. It is common in Turks and is associated with HLA-B5. There is suppressor T-cell and complement dysfunction and polymorphonuclear leucocyte motility. The antigen is unknown.

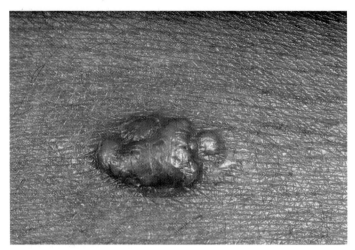

Fig. 21.3 Sarcoidosis

The lesions have a red–brown colour and are papules, nodules or plaques. There is no surface scaling because the granulomas are in the dermis and sometimes subcutaneous tissue but not in the epidermis. Compression of the skin with a glass slide (diascopy) often reveals an 'apple jelly' appearance. The diagnosis is by skin biopsy. This woman had pulmonary infiltrates on chest X-ray. The lesion responded to systemic steroids given for her concomitant lung pathology but could also have been treated with intralesional steroids.

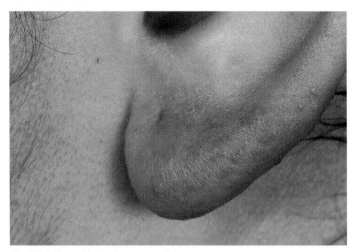

Fig. 21.4 Sarcoidosis (lupus pernio)

This variant affects the nose, ear lobes and cheeks (areas more vulnerable to cold and hence perniosis). There is a persistent purple infiltration and discoloration of the skin.

270

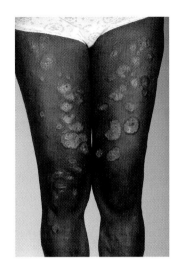

Fig. 21.5 Annular sarcoidosis
Lesions may be widespread and are
often annular in sarcoidosis. In
white skin they may be mauve or
in black skin red–brown in colour.

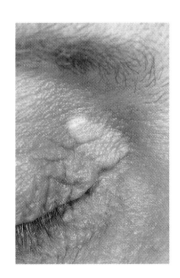

Fig. 21.6 Xanthelasma
There is a yellow, rather velvety
plaque in the inner canthus. These
are common and frequently the
lipid profiles are normal. They may
be treated by excision or destroyed
with cautery or trichloracetic acid
but they do tend to recur.

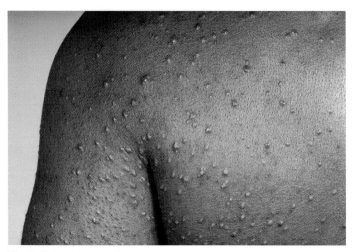

Fig. 21.7 Eruptive xanthomata
There are innumerable yellow papules and nodules. They erupt suddenly over a very short period of time. They are usually associated with hypertriglyceridaemia and high VLDL (very low density lipoproteins). They also occur in hyperlipidaemia secondary to diabetes mellitus as in this man.

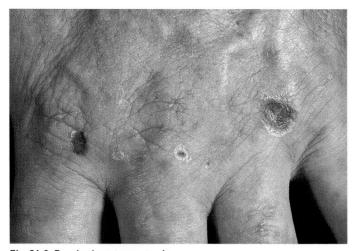

Fig. 21.8 Porphyria cutanea tarda
There is photosensitivity. The blisters and skin are generally fragile and break easily resulting in erosions and haemorrhagic scabs particularly on the back of the hands. The urine and stools should be examined for porphyrins. This variety is often associated with alcohol abuse or occasionally oestrogens and is due to a defective enzyme (uroporphyrinogen decarboxylase). The resultant accumulation of porphyrins may cause cirrhosis.

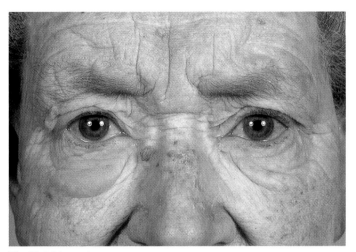

Fig. 21.9 Myxoedema
The appearance of the skin often provides the diagnosis before the symptoms of hypothyroidism which may not be complained of by the patient. There is a puffy non-pitting oedema around the eyes and a pallor and yellow tint to the skin due to anaemia and hypercarote-naemia. The hair is dry, brittle and tends to fall out. Treatment restores the facial appearance to normal.

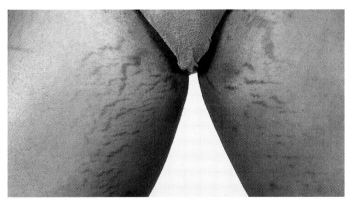

Fig. 21.10 Striae
Stretch marks such as these occur in Cushing's syndrome but the more common cause is the misuse of potent topical steroids.

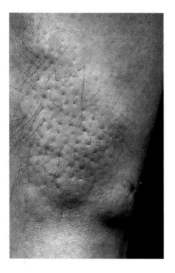

Fig. 21.11 Pretibial myxoedema
There is an infiltration of the dermis
with mucin giving rise to thickening
and oedema of the skin particularly
on the shins, due to excess
hyaluronic acid deposition in
Graves' disease. The hair follicle ori-
fices are patulous over the nodules
producing a peau d'orange appearance. There is hypertrichosis. It may
not appear until after treatment of
the hyperthyroidism. © Photograph
courtesy of St Mary's Hospital.

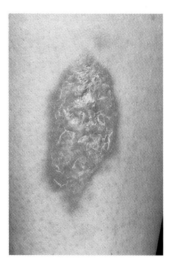

Fig. 21.12 Necrobiosis lipoidica
The plaque is very well defined.
Centrally there are yellowish areas
and peripherally a red or mauve
discoloration. Close inspection is
required to discern the telangiectasia. There is necrobiosis (destruction
of dermal collagen) surrounded by a
lymphocytic and granulomatous
infiltrate. There are changes of diabetic microangiopathy present in
diabetic cases.

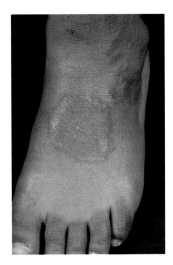

Fig. 21.13 Granuloma annulare
The lesion is ringed in shape and usually has a raised red non-scaling margin and a tendency to be flat and discoloured within. The dorsum of the foot is a common site.

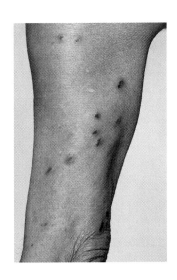

Fig. 21.14 Generalized pruritus
In generalized irritation of the skin secondary to a systemic cause, there are no signs of an underlying skin disorder, only scratch marks (excoriations).

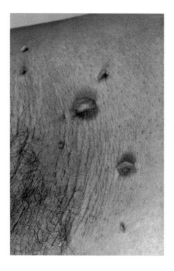

Fig. 21.15 Malignant acanthosis nigricans
There is a warty velvety thickening of the skin initially in the flexures but gradually more extensively with multiple skin tags and often seborrhoeic warts. This is very rare. This patient had an adenocarcinoma of the stomach. It is occasionally associated with lymphoma.

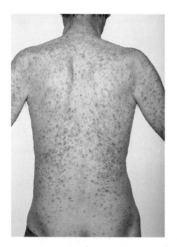

Fig. 21.16 Secondary deposits
This man had multiple hard purple nodules in his skin secondary to leukaemia. Secondary deposits from solid tumours are usually flesh coloured.

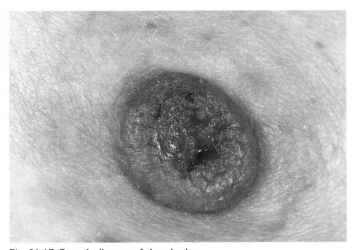

Fig. 21.17 Paget's disease of the nipple
There is a very well-defined plaque on the nipple which is red, eroded
and fissured. A biopsy established the diagnosis and an intraductal carcinoma was found on mammography.

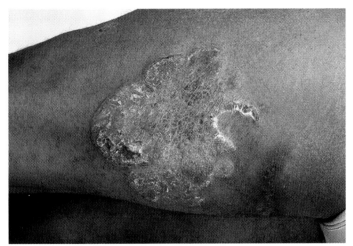

Fig. 21.18 Mycosis fungoides
As the patches progress the lesions thicken forming plaques and
tumours. Most patients have the condition for many decades without
this ever happening but 8% do progress and the lymph nodes and other
organs are involved. Treatment for these progressive T-cell tumours is
unsatisfactory.

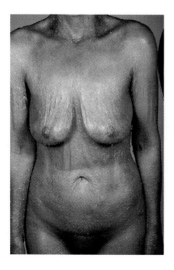

Fig. 21.19 Mycosis fungoides
Occasionally all the skin is involved
and the patient is erythrodermic.
There is usually lymphadenopathy
and circulating abnormal T cells
with large cerebriform nuclei
(Sézary cells). It is an intensely itchy
condition.

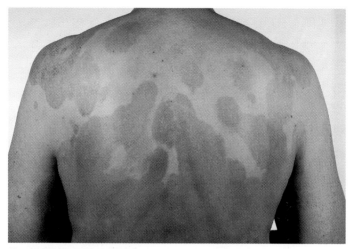

Fig. 21.20 Mycosis fungoides
The disorder is at various stages in its development. Some of the lesions
are a faint pink colour, others are red and some are a deep red colour.
The shapes vary: some are oval, others round and others triangular. The
sizes vary too. This patch/plaque stage responds very well to photochemotherapy or topical nitrogen mustard.

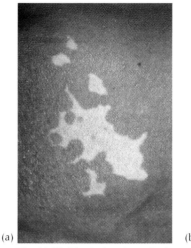 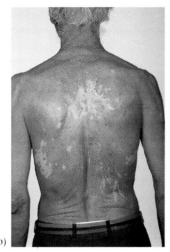

(a)   (b)

Fig. 21.21 Pityriasis rubra pilaris
The skin is virtually universally involved. The remarkable islands of
sparing are a clue to the diagnosis of this rare disorder which comes on
abruptly in the latter half of life. The skin has an orange or deep-red
colour. The cause is unknown but it may clear spontaneously after a
couple of years.

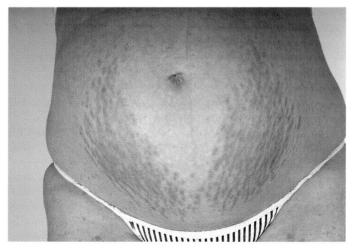

**Fig. 21.22 Polymorphic eruption of pregnancy (pruritic urticarial
papules and plaques of pregnancy—PUPPP)**
The condition begins in the abdominal striae in the last trimester of the
first pregnancy. There are urticarial lesions subsequently on the limbs
and body. The itching is so distressing that it may be an indication for
induction of labour. It does not occur in subsequent pregnancies.

22 Differential Diagnosis

The face

Inflammatory
- seborrhoeic eczema (Fig. 2.6)
- atopic eczema (Fig. 2.1)
- contact dermatitis
- psoriasis
- acne (Fig. 13.1)
- perioral and periorbital acne (Fig. 13.2)
- rosacea (Fig. 13.6)
- radiodermatitis

Bacterial infection
- impetigo
- erysipelas (Fig. 9.6)
- lupus vulgaris
- leprosy

Viral infection
- herpes simplex
- Kaposi's varicelliform eruption (Fig. 2.4)
- varicella (Fig. 11.2)
- herpes zoster
- vaccinia
- plane warts (Fig. 11.4)
- verruca vulgaris
- molluscum contagiosum (Fig. 11.5)
- measles
- fifth disease (Fig. 11.9)

Fungal infection
- tinea
- angular cheilitis

Infestation
- leishmaniasis

Congenital/developmental
- trichoepitheliomata
- tuberous sclerosus (Fig. 17.7)
- dermatosis papulosa nigra
- xeroderma pigmentosum

- basal cell naevus syndrome
- ulerythema oophryogenes

Reactive
- Sweet's disease
- angio-oedema

Drugs
- photosensitivity
- fixed drug eruption
- minocycline pigmentation

Immunological
- discoid lupus erythematosus (Fig. 18.12)
- dermatomyositis (Fig. 18.13)
- scleroderma
- morphoea
- alopecia areata
- vitiligo
- benign mucous membrane pemphigoid

Vascular
- lymphoedema
- amyloidosis

Systemic
- sarcoidosis (Fig. 21.3)
- xanthelasma (Fig. 21.6)
- myxoedema (Fig. 21.9)
- porphyria

Pigmentary disorders
- melasma (Fig. 15.1)
- localized ochronosis (Fig. 15.2)
- fixed drug eruption
- minocycline
- pityriasis alba (Fig. 15.3)

Psychological
- acne excoriée des jeunes filles
- dermatitis artefacta

Acute eruptions affecting the face
- impetigo
- erysipelas
- herpes simplex
- Kaposi's varicelliform eruption

- herpes zoster
- varicella
- vaccinia
- measles
- slapped cheek disease
- acute contact dermatitis
- photosensitivity

Solitary lesions on the face

Moles
- junctional naevus
- compound naevus (Fig. 6.11)
- intradermal naevus
- blue naevus
- juvenile melanoma

Red papules or nodules
- strawberry naevus
- pyogenic granuloma
- Kaposi's sarcoma

Yellow papules or plaques
- xanthelasma
- juvenile xanthogranuloma
- senile sebaceous hyperplasia

White or flesh-coloured papules or nodules
- calcifying epithelioma of Malherbe
- syringomata (Fig. 7.4)

Pigmented lesions
- solar lentigo
- seborrhoeic wart
- malignant melanoma (Fig. 8.12)
- pigmented basal cell carcinoma
- blue naevus

Warty, crusted or ulcerated lesions
- solar keratosis
- Bowen's disease
- keratoacanthoma (Fig. 8.11)
- squamous cell carcinoma (Fig. 8.8)
- basal cell carcinoma (Fig. 8.13)

The feet

Inflammatory
- podopompholyx (foot eczema)
- contact dermatitis
- juvenile plantar dermatosis
- psoriasis vulgaris
- pustular psoriasis
- keratoderma blenorrhagica (Fig. 3.10)
- lichen planus
- infantile acropustulosis

Bacterial infection
- secondary syphilis
- streptococcal infection

Viral infection
- hand, foot and mouth disease
- verruca

Fungal infection
- acute tinea
- chronic tinea pedis
- tinea incognito

Infestation
- scabies (Fig. 12.2)
- insect bites

Benign tumours
- eccrine poroma

Malignant tumours
- epithelioma cuniculatum
- acral lentiginous malignant melanoma

Developmental/congenital
- keratoderma
- punctate keratoderma
- epidermolysis bullosa

Vascular
- chilblains
- vasculitis
- gangrene
- capillaritis

Chapter 22

Systemic
* granuloma annulare (Fig. 21.11)

Trauma
* corns
* black-heel syndrome

Differential diagnosis of eruptions presenting acutely on the feet
* podopompholyx (foot eczema)
* contact dermatitis
* tinea
* streptococcal infection
* syphilis
* hand, foot and mouth disease
* vasculitis
* chilblains
* gangrene

Male genitalia

Inflammatory
* eczema
* psoriasis (Fig. 3.8)
* lichen planus (Fig. 5.5)
* lichen nitidus
* plasma cell balanitis of Zoon

Bacterial infection
* syphilis (chancre)
* secondary syphilis

Viral infection
* herpes simplex
* warts
* molluscum contagiosum
* Kaposi's sarcoma

Fungal infection
* candidosis

Infestation
* scabies (Fig. 12.2)

Naevi
* melanotic macules

Benign tumours
- pearly penile papules
- idiopathic calcinosis of the scrotum
- angiokeratoma

Malignant tumours
- Bowenoid papulosis
- genital Bowen's disease (Fig. 8.6)
- squamous cell carcinoma

Reactive/drugs
- erythema multiforme
- fixed drug eruption

Immunological
- vitiligo
- lichen sclerosus et atrophicus (Fig. 18.18)
- pemphigus

Vascular
- lymphoedema

Systemic
- Behçet's syndrome

Psychological
- dermatitis artefacta

The groin and pubic area in males

Inflammatory
- seborrhoeic eczema
- lichen simplex
- psoriasis
- lichen planus
- hidradenitis suppurativa (Fig. 13.5)

Bacterial infection
- erythrasma

Viral infection
- warts
- molluscum contagiosum
- herpes simplex

Fungal infection
- tinea cruris
- candidosis

Infestations
- pediculosis (Fig. 12.5)
- scabies

Drugs
- steroid-induced striae

Developmental
- Hailey–Hailey disease
- pseudo-acanthosis nigricans

Autoimmune
- pemphigus and other blistering disorders

Hair
- alopecia areata

Female genitalia

Inflammatory
- seborrhoeic eczema (Fig. 2.15)
- lichen simplex (Fig. 2.11)
- psoriasis
- lichen planus

Viral infection
- herpes simplex
- warts
- molluscum contagiosum

Fungal infection
- candidosis (Fig. 10.8)
- tinea cruris (see Fig. 10.6)

Infestation
- pediculosis pubis

Malignant skin tumours
- Bowen's disease
- squamous cell carcinoma (Fig. 8.5)
- extramammary Paget's disease

Drugs
• striae

Developmental
• Hailey–Hailey disease

Autoimmune
• lichen sclerosus et atrophicus (Fig. 18.17)

Hair
• alopecia areata

Pigmentation
• vulvovaginal melanosis

Systemic
• pyoderma gangrenosum

Psychological
• lichen simplex

The napkin (diaper) area in infants and children

Inflammatory
• napkin (diaper) dermatitis (Fig. 2.7)
• atopic eczema
• psoriasis
• seborrhoeic eczema
• post-inflammatory hypopigmentation

Infections
• bullous impetigo
• Kaposi's varicelliform eruption

Autoimmune
• chronic bullous dermatosis of childhood

Systemic
• Langerhan's cell histiocytosis

The hands

Inflammatory
• contact dermatitis (Fig. 2.2)

- pompholyx (Fig. 2.9)
- keratolysis exfoliativa
- psoriasis vulgaris (Fig. 3.6)
- pustular psoriasis (Fig. 3.4)
- lichen planus (Fig. 5.1)
- pityriasis rubra pilaris

Bacterial infection
- streptococcal hands
- gonococcaemia (Fig. 9.9)
- secondary syphilis

Viral infection
- warts
- hand, foot and mouth disease
- herpes simplex
- Orf (Fig. 11.10)

Fungal infection
- tinea (Figs. 10.5, 10.7)
- candida paronychia

Infestations
- larva migrans
- scabies (Fig. 12.1)

Congenital/developmental
- keratoderma

Reactive
- erythema multiforme

Immunological
- lupus erythematosus

Systemic
- palmar plane xanthomata
- carotenaemia
- palmar erythema
- hyperhidrosis

Skin disorders on the backs of the hands

Reactive/drug
- erythema multiforme (Fig. 19.6)
- photosensitivity

- fixed drug eruption (Fig. 19.13)
- steroid atrophy

Immunological
- chilblain lupus
- dermatomyositis (Fig. 18.14)
- scleroderma (Fig. 18.15)
- vitiligo

Vascular
- acrocyanosis

Systemic
- granuloma annulare
- sarcoidosis
- porphyria cutanea tarda (Fig. 21.8)
- carotenaemia
- plane xanthomata
- palmar erythema

Psychological
- dermatitis artefacta
- habit tic

Differential diagnosis of eruptions which may present acutely on the hands
- pompholyx
- contact dermatitis
- impetigo
- tinea
- herpes simplex
- acute paronychia
- photosensitivity
- fixed drug eruption
- erythema multiforme
- hand, foot and mouth disease (Fig. 11.8)
- lupus erythematosus
- streptococcal infection
- gonococcaemia
- orf (Fig. 11.10)

Differential diagnosis of solitary papules and nodules on the hands
- pyogenic granuloma
- eccrine poroma
- glomus tumour

- warts
- acral lentiginous melanoma
Especially on the backs of the hands:
- blue naevus
- solar lentigines
- solar keratosis (Fig. 8.1)
- Bowen's disease (Fig. 8.4)
- keratoacanthoma
- squamous cell carcinoma
- malignant melanoma

The torso

Inflammatory
- seborrhoeic eczema
- discoid eczema
- pityriasis rosea (Fig. 4.2)
- eczematide
- generalized eczema
- guttate psoriasis (Fig. 3.2)
- psoriasis vulgaris (Fig. 3.9)
- erythroderma
- acne (Fig. 13.3)
- pityriasis rubra pilaris (Fig. 21.21)
- lichen planus (Fig. 5.3)

Bacterial infection
- *Pseudomonas* folliculitis
- secondary syphilis (Fig. 9.11)

Viral infection
- varicella
- herpes zoster
- viral exanthems

Fungal infections
- tinea corporis
- pityriasis versicolor (Fig. 10.9)

Infestation
- eosinophilic folliculitis
- scabies

Reactive
- urticaria
- toxic erythema (Fig. 19.1)

- drug eruption
- erythema multiforme

Autoimmune
- pemphigoid (Fig. 18.4)
- pemphigus (Fig. 18.9)
- lupus erythematosus

Vascular
- pityriasis lichenoides (Fig. 20.7)

Developmental
- ichthyosis (Fig. 17.1)
- Darier's disease (Fig. 17.3)
- von Recklinghausen's disease (Fig. 17.6)

Systemic
- sarcoidosis
- non-Hodgkin's lymphoma
- mycosis fungoides (Fig. 21.20)
- neoplastic deposits (Fig. 21.14)
- spider naevi
- amyloid
- urticaria pigmentosum
- xanthomata (Fig. 21.7)

Differential diagnosis of some eruptions presenting acutely, especially on the torso

- pityriasis rosea (Fig. 4.2)
- guttate psoriasis (Fig. 3.2)
- secondary syphilis
- folliculitis (bacterial)
- varicella
- herpes zoster
- viral exanthems
- urticaria
- toxic erythema
- drug eruptions
- erythema multiforme
- staphylococcal scalded skin syndrome

Annular eruptions

Differential diagnosis of eruptions that are often annular

Inflammatory
• psoriasis
• annular lichen planus
• annular seborrhoeic dermatitis

Infections
• tinea
• leprosy
• syphilis
• Lyme disease

Skin cancer
• basal cell carcinoma

Reactive
• drug eruptions
• urticaria

Immunological
• lupus erythematosus

Systemic
• mycosis fungoides
• figurate erythemas
• granuloma annulare
• sarcoidosis

Index

Note: Page numbers in **bold** refer to tables, page numbers in *italic* refer to figures.

WITHDRAWN
FROM STOCK
QMUL LIBRARY